MW01254003

Healthcare

It Mostly Works

What You Should Know

by

Furley Lumpkin
with
Chris Carrington

RoseDog Books
PITTSBURGH, PENNSYLVANIA 15222

ISBN: 978-1-4349-9628-2
Printed in the United States of America

First Printing

Original Copyright 2008

For more information or to order additional books, please contact:
RoseDog Books
701 Smithfield Street
Pittsburgh, Pennsylvania 15222
U.S.A.
1-800-834-1803
www.rosedogbookstore.com

Dedication

This book is dedicated to Red and Sibyl Lumpkin.

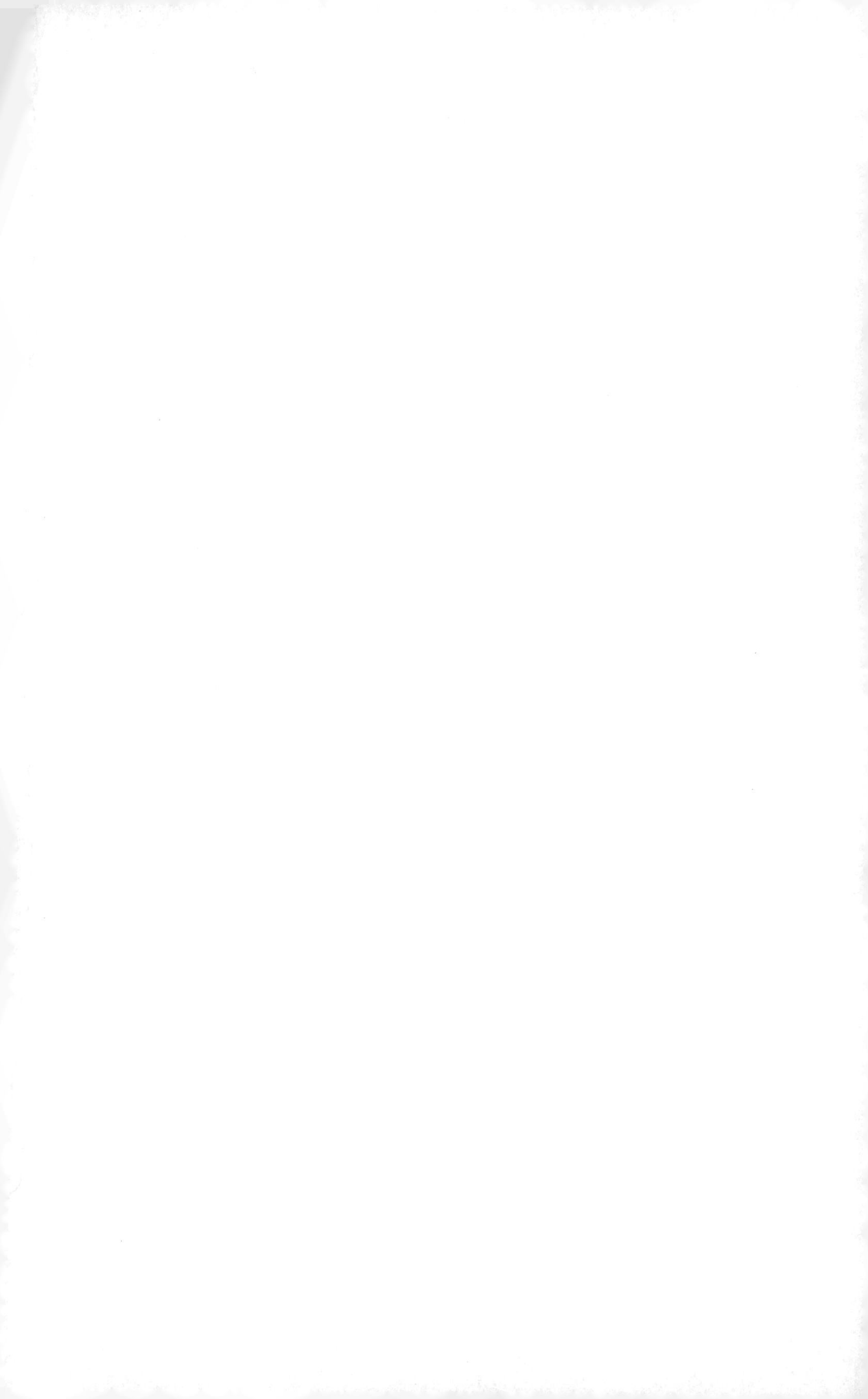

TABLE OF CONTENTS

Foreword

There are few businesses that offer the opportunity to be of service in the way a hospital does. Technology is changing the practice of medicine in dramatic ways, both positive and negative. There are those that are comfortable with the evolution of technology and there are those that are not. There are those that say technology will reduce errors and improve outcomes—and they are right, if it is used correctly and built upon accurate information, and more importantly, is equally easy to use whether you are a technology-averse person or not. We are all smart in different ways and the most caring nurse or doctor may find the forced format of computer commands to be confusing, making what is designed to be a life-saving tool into something altogether different.

The best illustration of this was during the hospitalization of my—Furley's— brother. The ICU nurse entered the room with a computer on wheels (sometimes called a COW) and then pulled out a paper towel to write down his vitals. When asked why she did this, she responded that she didn't like to type things in front of other people and she would do it later. When this particular hospital's corporate office introduced an Electronic Medical Record by mandate from a thousand miles away, this nurse was not in their thought process.

So now when you cross the threshold into a hospital, regardless of your role, you should have a realistic understanding of what is happening behind the scenes—operationally, financially, legally, technologically, and managerially. Understanding these issues is important as a family member of someone who is ill or as an employee of a hospital who is hired to provide care to the patient, because in the end the outcomes are not the responsibility of one person, but the responsibility of a very large team of people, many of whom you will never meet.

Ultimately, a hospital is a business where those of us with illnesses or injuries go to find hope. But in truth, it is a corporate entity with decision makers that may have agendas that are more relevant to their future career moves than to your care. As we researched the material, we realized that we were writing for those that will take care of others when they are not able to take care of themselves. Our goal was to provide patients, family members, healthcare providers and IT professionals with a common frame of reference for a field that all of us will experience in one way or another.

Chapter 1

The Last One Hundred Years

If we are fortunate to live longer, healthier lives, as scientists predict, then our involvement in the healthcare system, as it exists today and into the future, is going to be very important. To imagine how different the practice of medicine will be in another hundred years is easier when we reflect upon how different the world is now from how it was a century ago. In the late 1800s and early 1900s, our economy was undergoing dramatic changes. We were moving from a largely rural population and a farm-based economy that emphasized self-reliance to more of an urban-based population that made it's living in industrial and manufacturing areas. The automobile and telephone were invented, the Wright Brothers took their first flight, and eventually these developments became widely used throughout society. This growth served to force our nation to evolve into a national community.

As our healthcare system changed in the last one hundred years, our methods of payment for medical care and the cost of medical care have changed. It was essential to increase the accessibility of healthcare to our citizens as we became a more urbanized society and Congress determined that it was important to provide healthcare insurance through employers, as had been successfully provided to the military during World War II. The health of our population is fundamental to economic well-being and even to our national security. Congress enacted incentives in the form of tax breaks for employers who provided health insurance to their employees. These tax incentives remain in place today. According to http://taxfoundation.org/, it is "the largest preference in the tax code with an estimated 2006 value of roughly $126 billion."

This was a successful plan and it is important to understand that our current system provides health coverage to six out of seven people in the United States, or approximately 253,000,000 people, largely because of the federal government's post-World War II tax incentives. This is assuming an estimated population of nearly 300,000,000 based upon recent estimates by the United States Census Bureau. One criterion for a good job is still considered the provision of high quality health insurance, in order to provide a safety net when catastrophic illnesses or accidents occur.

The cost of supplying this healthcare has grown exponentially as coverage provided through employers has become more pervasive. This increase is the result of covering a broader base of our population, including those with chronic conditions. Treatment options that have improved substantially while becoming more complex, diagnostic tools that have developed resulting in earlier detection of once fatal conditions, and the higher cost-of-living have all served to drive up the cost of healthcare. In addition, physicians and patients learned that there were ways to get coverage for elective procedures by justifying it as a "medical necessity," sometimes when that wasn't completely the case. To counterbalance this effort, insurance companies became increasingly aggressive in their procedures to ensure proper utilization.

As the costs associated with employer-paid health insurance increased and insurance was provided to a greater part of the population, the role of the physician caring for you began having more comprehensive oversight, swinging to the business side of healthcare, away from the exclusive domain of the physician. This occurred primarily to keep costs down, where it was deemed necessary, and to avoid inappropriate use. While the medical side of healthcare has been slower than the business side in adopting technology because it hasn't historically been driven by the same financial incentives, it has inched into the actual delivery of medical care over the preceding decades.

The interdependence between technology and healthcare requires constant change, including changes in the way your relationship with your physician is acted upon. Personal phone calls are no longer always needed when a recorded system can provide you with test results for routine medical tests, such as blood sugar tests or when an e-mail can trigger a physician to authorize a prescription refill. These small technological advantages can free up the time of your physician or their staff and allow them to concentrate on more immediate personal care delivery. It can also help keep costs down.

The medical community is filled with people who want to help other people. They combine the best of the practice of medicine with generous and kind hearts that help us through some of our most difficult times and some of our most joyous experiences.

One such example was Dr. S. H. "Bud" Dryden in Austin, Texas. My parents met Dr. Dryden in 1952, shortly after moving to Austin, and until their deaths, my mother and father always considered Dr. Dryden to be their doctor. They never accepted medical advice from someone not approved and recommended by Dr. Dryden. He was the only doctor my father felt comfortable talking to, possibly because my father never felt like Dr. Dryden was trying to impress him with how smart he was—he spoke in plain, understandable terms. He was a friend, someone who spoke to you when he saw you and remembered you. He asked how you were and he meant it. He made house calls when needed because it was best for you.

In his later years, when my mother was ill, she called Dr. Dryden to get his personal endorsement of the treatment she was pursuing. Knowing her condition was terminal, he gave her just the right amount of information and comfort. This trust was something that was built over a lifetime of helping my family through different medical and personal crises. My favorite story occurred in the 1960s when my mother's sisters were all having hysterectomies for a variety of reasons, partially because doctors recommended them for women of that "certain age." My mother had just turned forty and went to Dr. Dryden for his opinion about whether or not she should consider a hysterectomy. He responded with, "Hell, Sibyl, if you need one, I need one," and that was the end of that discussion.

Technology will not replace these essential relationships, but it can be used as a tool to augment this type of care that any of us may need at some point in the future. The American healthcare system delivers some of the best outcomes in the world built upon the work of people like Dr. Dryden and his nurse, Ethel, but the world of medicine is no longer limited to these relationships. Now when you walk into a physician's office, you may only see the physician and receptionist, but the room is crowded with unseen people who are directly involved in your care. It is no longer just the doctor and you, or the nurse and you.

The immutable core of healthcare is built on a foundation of relationships over which the physician applies expertise based upon their historical knowledge of you and your condition, in combination with their knowledge of what works and the medical tools they have available. Technology is now one of these tools. Successful healthcare must start with a relationship between the patient, their family, and the nurse or physician. Understanding the wide variety of people throughout the hospital involved in the delivery of tools and technology the medical professionals will use is important because each of these people will be in the exam room with the physician, even if they are unseen. The people who provided the physician the computer, the programmer who built the Computerized Physician Order Entry system or Electronic Health Record, the people who design and manage the computer network are all in the exam room with your physician in one form or another. If you don't believe this, next time you visit your physician just count the number of computers you see as you walk through their office suite. Now imagine that none of them work or that none of them can connect to one another. The interdependency of medicine and technology will become clear.

Chapter 2

Why is technology personally important?

Healthcare is the subject of considerable political rhetoric, and few political issues have as much impact on our personal lives as the international discussion on the topic. Healthcare has changed as technology and research have created new diagnostic tools, and the availability of information has grown exponentially over the last few decades. Entering a new century, physicians collaborate instantaneously with colleagues across the globe through a variety of media—voice teleconferences, video conferencing, and remote learning tools on the Web, to name a few. One of the greatest challenges faced by physicians and other medical professionals is deciding how to use this information and finding a filter for the information so they can focus their efforts on what is relevant. This is one issue behind the rapid expansion of Computerized Physician Order Entry (CPOE) systems and Electronic Health (or Medical) Records (EHR). These systems will allow physicians to respond to your needs more quickly and from remote sites, regardless of where you are, if the need arises.

In an emergency the ultimate benefit is clear, as your personal physician may be part of the team working to save your life without leaving their office. Technology will improve access to care in remote places of our nation and will help medical professionals expand their practice to parts of our planet in great need of what is one of our national assets—a truly outstanding community of medical professionals and researchers. This will place a demand on technology infrastructure between the hospital, the physician's office, and your home. Whether you live in the heart of a major metropolitan community or in a rural community, the availability of this technology will inevitably play a major role in your future health and the delivery of your healthcare.

The provision of your medical care will begin to require that you become informed about your care and options in ways that you have not in the past. However, the truth is that when placed in a situation requiring emergency care or assistance due to a severe chronic illness that impairs our ability to think clearly, we are at the mercy of the medical community. But our health is not just dependent upon our doctor's knowledge and his or her access to information in general, but on access to our specific conditions and medical history. Regardless of how averse you are to technology, your medical record is something that must be accessible by healthcare professionals in a wide variety of unanticipated circumstances.

Besides improving our clinical outcomes, the speed at which researchers can communicate—the ability to sort through billions of records in seconds—will help pinpoint virus outbreaks will help save lives. However, because of the focus on the information available through technology, it is going to be increasingly important for the patient to communicate their experience to the physician or nurse. We cannot sit passively, allowing a healthcare provider to make recommendations at a time when we may have just been given the worst news of our lives and our mind is spinning.

It is going to be equally important that medical professionals develop realistic expectations about the performance of technology that is designed to help them make better decisions. They must recommit themselves to the initial goal of medicine—treating people, not cases. Technology is a tool for this treatment, but can never be allowed to subjugate the physician or nurse's responsibility. It is going to be essential that the technologist clearly define what these realistic expectations should be and share a commitment to providing high performing technology infrastructure and devices.

Ultimately, medicine is about people treating people. Technology is only a tool for that treatment; each patient is different, each nurse is different, and every hospital is different. Each circumstance must be approached individually. At the beginning of the twenty-first century, healthcare is engaged in adopting the use of technology and in the course of doing so, exposing weaknesses and reliability issues that were heretofore unimportant. In the past, who cared if e-mail was unavailable for an hour or if you couldn't get to your favorite shopping site? Now, whether you are the patient, the caregiver, a medical professional, or a hospital administrator the availability of electronic information is an issue that is very different when applied in the actual practice of medicine.

Chapter 3

The Challenges Before Us

Illness or injury rarely happens on a schedule or when it is most convenient for you to get to your physician. The information stored about you in one hospital or at your physician's office may not be readily available to those who are treating you in an emergency situation. Technological advances such as the development of electronic health records (EHR) are often praised as a solution and they are correctly extolled as such. However, they only work if the information about you is available. There are many different types of EHR applications developed by companies such as Epic, Eclipsys, GE Centricity, Medetech, etc. The information in any one of these applications is not automatically transferable from one system to the other. In fact, they are competitors who do not design their systems for interoperability with each other. This is important to note, particularly if you may find yourself in a hospital being treated by a physician that doesn't know you. You must take the initiative or have someone with you who will take this initiative. More importantly, we must demand that the flow of information between various hospitals and physicians be addressed in some manner.

Anytime you face a health issue, equip yourself with as much information as you can about the condition, the treatment environment, and the people treating you. Make sure your physicians and nurses know that you are informed and make sure they are informed of all your medications—prescription and non-prescription—any previous abnormalities in tests, chronic conditions, and your family history. Most importantly, assuming you are in control, never let them do or give you anything without a clear purpose. If you are unable to speak for yourself, have an advocate to make sure that your care is understood. Outcomes are almost always improved with a personal advocate.

A very important step for all Americans is to challenge the leaders of software, technology, and insurance organizations to create a universal, fully portable tool that can be carried in your pocket, wallet, or purse that contains all of your medical information. It is vital to the medical outcome that this device can be read by medical professionals at any point in time and works regardless of the type of computer being used. Security of the information can be provided using biometrics (fingerprint or retinal scanning) for access validation and it should not be downloadable except when permitted by two forms of authentication. Ideally, the information would use open source software and contain information such as existing diagnoses, medications, family medical history, and dental records. It might be a credit card device that is swiped or a portable USB flash drive downloaded by the pharmacist at the point of purchase so that the physician is aware of all your medications. The names of medications are not easy to remember. What most people recall is the frequency we take the pill(s), maybe the color and shape, and lastly, the amount. A tool of this type would be very valuable to treating physicians.

We don't usually prepare for a trip to the emergency room and you may be unable to communicate information that could save your life. Rarely does a physician that already knows you—and whether you have had a propensity for any type of action, reaction, or behavior—treat you. For your safety, there needs to be a uniform, standardized way for your medical history to follow your body. They (the doctors, nurses, and paramedics) certainly don't always know what medications you are on, and which might interact with the planned treatment protocol. They simply don't have a frame of reference for who you were before you arrived in the ER, the surgery suite, the ICU, or anywhere else they might be treating you. For this reason, a device that carries all your information is critical for your well-being.

Technology can enhance patient care by reducing risks associated with the lack of information; it will address the "low hanging fruit" so that the medical professionals can focus their efforts on the issues at hand. The portability of this information by creating a tool that can be used with any electronic medical record will avoid the time-consuming discussions needed to create the standards for an EMR. Placing markers that identify the location of core information that can be easily read by any application should be an easy accomplishment. Our ingenuity is limited only by our imagination.

Chapter 4

Technology: "The New Scalpel"

There are three parts to the availability of electronic medical information. The first is the application itself. The second is the transport medium or how the information travels from location A to location B and the third is the end-user device where the information is received, read, acted upon and sometimes initiated. The status of each of these areas must be identified before widespread implementation of any application.

The Application

The most important element of any technology application in healthcare is that the design of the application must be intuitive and easily usable, with logical indicators when additional information is available in other areas. It needs to be searchable in a way that is as simple as the wide variety of Internet search engines such as Google. The physician or nurse should be able to input a simple question when in the patient's electronic chart and get answers back rapidly. Questions such as, "What medication is this patient on?" should be searchable within the Electronic Medical Record (EMR).

There are many different types of EMR systems, with as many versions as there are models of cars. You may have a Ford, but you need to know if it is a Taurus or an F150 to determine what it is capable of doing. If you are a physician with privileges at multiple hospitals, you may have to know a variety of systems, and unfortunately, they are not as simple as driving as a car. They are all different and this is the central reason behind a need for standardization.

Perhaps most importantly, each medical provider using the system should be able to customize the information that is available so that it may be viewed in the most expeditious manner possible. When confronted with performance issues with a system, technologists will often say that the application is working as designed, negating the experience of the individual. Their job may be to force user acceptance of slower performance, or to drive behavioral or learning changes that will make the system viable in the future. Perhaps their motivation is to make sure they keep their job by avoiding the statement that the application needs to be fixed because it would take time and money that isn't available. Any time a technologist is told that a system has performance issues and responds with, "the system is working as designed," the medical provider should insist the design be re-visited.

The Transport Medium (aka The Network)

The second part of electronic information is the network, and this is where most of the risks of failure reside. Local Area Networks (LANs) are used throughout an organization to transmit data. These LANs connect through a series of devices that are located generally within 300 feet from a device called a switch. This distance limitation is based upon the type of cabling used. These devices are homed back to a main distribution frame in the building where the network routers are located, and these are connected to the data center that houses the servers where the application actually resides. A Wide Area Network (WAN) connects multiple buildings together to one common data center. Many people would offer the suggestion that the equipment should just go wireless, but the unfortunate reality is that current technology still requires the wireless access point to be connected to the hardwired network. Your laptop computer may be wireless, but the access point in the building isn't. Equally important, these networks have limitations in terms of capacity that could cause delays in the speed at which the information you are seeking is received. Another factor affecting the speed of these networks is the number of users accessing the servers simultaneously.

The Device

The third part of electronic information is the device that the person is using. If they are accessing the information from a PC or a Mac, there are compatibility issues that must be assessed. Just because something worked on one PC, doesn't mean it will work or perform as required on another PC, particularly if the two PCs use different operating systems, different browsers, or have a different set of updates for these. There are many different operating systems for computers and hand-held devices, and they change more frequently than a Southern California driver changes lanes. Few hospitals have forecasted the need for IT capital more than a couple of years out with any degree of accuracy, simply because the technology is obsolete before it is delivered. Equally important, there are nuances as to how to use this technology that will differ from device to device, adding a layer of complexity that didn't exist when all you had to do was turn the page in the chart (assuming everything was filed correctly).

The net result is that performance issues are inevitable and each one must be taken seriously. Testing should never be done in the production environment, but upgrades should be able to be implemented in a production environment without downtime. The only accurate way to validate that the system is functioning as designed is to have a major investment in a technology lab with constant efforts made to stress test a system in a design configuration similar to your own, leading back to a mock up of the environment technologically, as well as physically. There needs to be a "Development Lab" for architectural and physical functionality, as well as technology. Whether this is done in a university environment, internally, or by an independent third party is irrelevant—it is action that must be taken to achieve a medical grade technology network. The best candidates for this are likely medical or nursing school students, and perhaps this needs to become a major part of the curriculum.

Computer Speed vs. Blink Speed

Various channels through which information flows to the caregiver are a remarkable development in technology. The technologists will present this as a great asset, which it is, but if there is any delay from the point of accessing the application where the information is stored, the medical community will consider it to be unsatisfactory, which it also is. Life happens at "blink speed." The capacity of the human brain to process information is different from the capacity of a network, a PC, a handheld device, or a server. As long as our brain is distracted with activities related to getting the information we want or need, we feel like we are making progress. If we make the request electronically and then have a delay in the response, we feel as if there is interference to accomplishing our task.

In the past, if you were dictating medical notes for the paper chart, you were active. If you were reviewing a patient's chart, you could actively control the speed at which you reviewed it. In the EMR environment, you forfeit that control, resulting in persistent frustration between IT and the caregiver. The true measure of a successful IT project is acceptance as a result of ease of use. A successful CIO must be able to communicate in these human terms. Anyone in a leadership position in IT must first be able to communicate effectively to his or her overall user community. The true test of this ability is when the user community can translate what they've been told into an operational understanding of the system and issues.

Chapter 5

Who Creates "The New Scalpel?"

The tools used by physicians and nurses in your treatment have moved beyond the physical tools—scalpels, IVs, needles, sutures, etc. The physicians now must contend with electronic tools for decision support—electronic information that predicts the effectiveness of the treatment they are recommending. When facing our own mortality, there are as many responses as there are individuals facing the inevitable. It is this unique combination of our response and the caregivers' skills that determines how best to approach a medical situation, but this is also informed by the selection of technology tools with which the physician or nurse may or may not be completely comfortable. In addition to this, they may be asked to justify their proposed treatment to an administrator who is equally concerned with the bottom line or who has a serious risk aversion issue.

The true reality is that the skills that make an excellent physician or nurse are not necessarily those that are used to develop technological tools. There is truth in the perception that many technologists often have weak interpersonal skills, particularly in those situations where urgency is needed and high emotions may prevail—like in the hospital. The twenty-first century is not the first time in the history of humanity that we face two colliding skill sets with similar goals, but completely different points of origin. The challenge is to allow these two mindsets to merge over time and not force it on those who see the patient face-to-face, when he has tears streaming down his face because he is a forty-year-old man with a diagnosis that might prevent him seeing his children grown. Ultimately, medicine is humanity at its best and we must equip it with tools that are supportive of the *persons* involved in the care choices. It is more important to have standardized tools than to have the unrealistic expectation that care procedures can be completely standardized and driven by technology without regard for the unique experience of each patient or the unique knowledge of their caregiver. Tools must be created based upon reasonable standards, which can reasonably be expected to be in use for ten years without becoming antiquated—tools that will fully function regardless of the type of device used to access them and which will help keep the cost of healthcare manageable, while improving the availability of patient centric information.

The lifecycle of technology is relatively short—three to five years. The economics of healthcare are such that this speed of hardware change is a tool in providing medical care, much like a scalpel, and it is unsustainable over the long haul. Manufacturers of hardware and developers of software need to focus on a longer life cycle for their product with a lower dependency on updates. The concept that "it mostly works" or we will fix it in the next revision, is not acceptable in healthcare.

According to an Associated Press article by Jessica Mintz, which appeared in the *Austin American Statesman* on April 14, 2008, "Microsoft Corp.'s operating systems run most personal computers around the globe and are a cash cow for the world's largest software manufacturer." In the same paper on the same date, an article was reprinted from *The Dallas Morning News* written by Andrew D. Smith. It quotes Kent Novak, Vice President of Texas Instruments' medical and high-reliability business unit as saying, "Medical is already one of our faster-growing business units and things only get more exciting the further out you look." Corporate America views healthcare as a very deep financial growth pool.

The misunderstanding is that corporate America also continues to push for healthcare reform and wants to reduce their share of the costs to cover their own employees. They believe that this can be done without achieving longer product life cycles while maintaining pricing models that view healthcare as part of their "cash cow." The technology used in other businesses, such as oil companies and banks, is often the same that is used by hospitals. They need to address this within their own organizations, and hospitals should mandate that these vendors commit to a longer product life cycle, with fewer updates required. This will mean a higher level of quality assurance for products to be considered medical grade.

This leads to the question of who are the technologists that often are involved in making the decisions about what systems are used in hospitals. Most hospitals have created a position in their "C Suite"—Chief Executive Officer (CEO), Chief

Operating Officer (COO), Chief Financial Officer (CMO), Chief Medical Officer (CMO), Chief Nursing Officer (CNO), etc.—to take care of the technology needs of the hospital. The Chief Information Officer (CIO) is perhaps more important than anyone other than your physician or nurse. They are responsible for the computer systems, the network, the PCs, the servers, and the data storage devices that are used by the medical professionals who take care of you. Your doctor is not alone with you in the exam room, the operating room, or any time they are interacting with you. You should know who else is participating in your care, directly or indirectly.

Every physician and nurse will have a unique set of requirements, so the role of the CIO is to negotiate the potential minefield of "business owner" needs and to help ensure that the needs are prioritized, to minimize complaints and exposure to risks. This often pits the "business" departments of the hospital against the "clinical" areas. It would be incorrect to assume that all needs are going to be met or that politics, vendor preference, and favoritism for one staff member over another doesn't enter into the decision.

The CIO may report to any of the aforementioned "C Suite" personnel (CEO, CFO, COO, CMO, CNO). By now, you've ascertained that there are a lot of "chiefs" in healthcare. To take the metaphor one step further, remember, there is only one "medicine man." The role of a CIO is very difficult to fill and has a high failure rate, often resulting in the joke that the phrase CIO stands for "career is over." Regardless of the reporting structure and lip service to the contrary, the administrative leadership of most hospitals just wants the CIO "to make the bad thing go away," as the other administrative leaders' knowledge of technology is often limited to turning on their computers and accessing their e-mail or daily schedules.

Filling the role of CIO has not been met with overwhelming success. The first requirement of a CIO must be to explain complex technology in a way that is understood by everyone involved in the process. They also need to explain the risks associated with each option under consideration and accurately set expectations. The ideal CIO is not restricted hierarchically, but solicits, values, and respects the opinion of all staff with whom they work, throughout the organization, as well as any input the patients or community may have. They must be actively involved in the life of the medical center, viewed as a service-oriented person, and always willing to listen. Most importantly, they must be collaborative in nature and should pay attention to all of their constituents and their direct reports.

Many of us have seen scalpels, at least on television. The technological advancements that continue to occur must be considered to be a similar tool that the providers of care will use. The challenge will be to make these providers comfortable with it. Their view of the tool is limited to the computer in front of them and they have an expectation that as soon as they enter a piece of information it is automatically dispersed throughout the caregiving universe. This is largely due to the failure of technologists to properly set expectations. Why are the expectations not correctly set? Perhaps if the caregivers knew the reality of what they were getting, the adoption of this technology would take longer, much longer. Too often the philosophy of "it mostly works" is exactly the operating philosophy of the technologists.

Chapter 6

Technology: Oops, the scalpel broke

During my mother's illness, we became concerned that her cancer had spread to her brain, as is the normal path for small cell carcinoma. We were not certain if this was the problem or if there was another issue unrelated to the cancer, so we spoke with her oncologist and scheduled an MRI. We followed the MRI with a brief trip to her sisters' house. The trip took great effort on her part to appear completely normal, but she didn't let on to anyone how serious her condition was, although most knew.

When we returned home, I called to see if the results of the MRI had been received. The doctor didn't have them, so I followed up with the company that did the MRI. A supervisor told me that they had been implementing a new PACS (Picture Archiving and Communications System) for the MRI and had a failure after the visit. She had lost not only the original, but she confessed that they didn't have a backup procedure in place.

Although it was naïve, I held the expectation that the computerized records needed for the care of my family were given a priority that was higher than just about any other computer record. The reality turned out to be that the business decisions regarding the system were made outside of the clinical realm by management or leadership. It was frustrating to know that a simple decision to go live without a backup procedure in place caused so much anguish.

We take for granted that these systems are designed to avoid a failure and should be very redundant with multiple methods of accessing the same information, but it begs the question, "What do we take for granted when we enter the hospital?" Does the IT department understand that they are impacting patient lives and each installation is not just another "business case?" Any system implemented in a healthcare setting that does not have viable backups, including how the information will be accessed in a system or device failure, should be reconsidered. Any executive that allows funds to be spent on a system without having certain knowledge that backups are incorporated into the plan should consider whether or not they have lost their focus.

Their challenge is that often the IT Manager will present a budget for X, long before understanding the business needs of the care provider. When these additional business needs are identified, IT managers often identify it as a change in scope and request large funding increases. A major HMO experienced just this in their implementation of an electronic record, as did another well-known hospital that allowed a CIO to build a computerized physician order entry system, even when his standing joke was that he "didn't like being around sick people" and avoided patient floors in the hospital. It was this same CIO that jokingly said on many occasions "Hey, it mostly works," should be the motto for IT. It sounds bizarre, but this kind of attitude exists and may kill people. Would you get on an airplane if the pilot announced that we were cleared for takeoff since the plane "mostly works?"

It's interesting to note that in the *Los Angeles Times* on September 4, 2007, Tami Abdollah quotes Ken Ritchart, assistant commissioner in the Office of Information and Technology with U. S. Customs and Border Protection, as saying "everything has been moved up. We recognize the fact that having folks sit on airplanes for hours is not acceptable, so we have to look at new procedures..." Mr. Ritchart is referring to an outage involving the computer systems at the Los Angeles International Airport on August 11, which continued unresolved for several days. Is this acceptable on the runway of an airport? Is it more or less acceptable in the ICU or surgery suite? It depends upon your perspective.

I believe that all healthcare IT decisions made by a project sponsor should be based upon the perspective of the patient—the person laying on the hospital bed/stretcher/gurney. At a minimum, when agencies are charged with monitoring the performance of a hospital or medical group, or providing licensure for their facilities, they should ask questions and not be dazzled by the "techno-speak" of the HIT managers and leaders. If technology questions cannot be described in terms that are easily understood by all audiences, those charged with implementing the system or application do not understand the operational needs.

In the "C-Suite," success is most likely measured by how little they hear about IT, and the executive leadership of the organization has not thought of asking IT to produce an executive summary of backup procedures for the hospital leadership. Perhaps they avoid this discussion because they don't want an hour-long presentation that doesn't make sense to them. As long as they can access the Internet, Intranet, and their e-mail, they are happy campers with IT. They can tell you where they stand on budget and awards the organization has won long before they can articulate fact-based confidence that backup procedures are in place.

Technology's share of available capital funding is growing rapidly and some forecasts indicate that the healthcare community cannot sustain these costs or the rate of change. Projects that are over budget and/or lack the acceptance of the end-user community are swept under the rug, used for a short interim period, and then discarded. If an unacceptable system is forcibly installed, the staff will create shadow procedures to get around the system. Everyone knows you need a good billing system, but if it breaks, you can send a corrected bill. The patient care arena does not allow for "do-overs." The delivery of patient care is integral to a fully integrated, implemented, accepted, and high-performing technology network. The new scalpel must be a precision, medical grade instrument.

When challenged to do so, the basis for the review of application performance should be that the user is right. In some respects maybe we are getting back to the point where "the customer is always right," where urgent communications between providers of care are done person-to-person rather than via e-mail.

The path of technology implementations is paved with the stories of failures caused by mandating support against the wishes and expectations of caregivers. However, this is the paradox: there is a point at which the support may need to be mandated, but only when the requests are unreasonable and the users know that their concerns are well documented and will be addressed in the future. This requires the delicate balancing of issues and considerable skill in making sure that all constituents feel heard, are heard, and are kept informed about what is being done to address their concerns.

An organization's ability to address user problems within an application both rapidly and honestly will determine the future ability of the organization to secure support—financial and operational—to implement new systems, equipment, and applications. This is the point where the importance of the choice of a CIO is most clearly demonstrated. Their ability to listen to their colleagues throughout the organization and to discard internal politics and publicly allow doubt is crucial to the process of a successful implementation. There are lively discussions everywhere about the criteria for selecting a CIO, but the first must be their willingness to listen and lead. You can hire technologists, but leaders are far rarer. The question to ask is, "Who do I trust to tell me the truth when we are in failure mode?"

When an organization's IT infrastructure is in failure mode and the organization is relying heavily upon electronic information, it will very likely have an impact on lives. All hospitals have a set of Policies & Procedures (P&Ps) that are the rules documented for all staff to follow. Are these easily available and is the staff quizzed on them? Wouldn't it be awful if the only test of the staff's understanding of the P&Ps were when they made an error in your treatment or in responding to your need while you are incapacitated?

CHAPTER 7

THE HOSPITAL INFORMATION NETWORK

Why is speed on the network so important? Have you ever accessed the Internet and had to wait for something to pop up on your screen? This happens on a hospital computer network too, but the consequences may be more than delayed e-mail—they are delayed care. Imagine that you are a patient in distress and access to the network is slow, or worse, it's completely unavailable. The organizations responsible for licensure of medical clinics and accreditation of hospitals should incorporate a thorough review of hospital networks and require self-reporting of outages, downtimes (planned or unplanned), and medical staff complaints regarding these issues. The availability of information is an exceptionally important element of the caregiving process.

Fortunately, hospitals are recognizing this and are focusing on the ability of staff to access information. Few hospitals measure accessibility of information all the way to the actual computer, instead they measure the "availability" of the application, but rarely correlate this to the secure accessibility of the data to all providers of care. There are few standardized measurements for this type of job competency in place in most major medical centers, leaving much ambiguity in the meaning of reports. Accreditation boards, the Department of Health Services, or any other licensing or permitting board should require hospitals to provide documentation of the accessibility and ability of the staff to access this information. Hospitals should be required to administer tests and report the results on all major clinical systems in place, and when the staff is not fully able to utilize the system, don't penalize the staff, but take the system off-line until it can be used without risk to patients. Using this information must be second nature, just like reading the paper and turning to the section you find most interesting.

The medical community has a low tolerance for anything that doesn't go according to plan. Beyond the issue of multiple systems being used for clinical information—forcing physicians and nurses to use them—is the matter of the reliability of these systems. The systems are not monolithic and the information is actually comprised of multiple layers, as described in the preceding chapter. A failure in any of these layers can result in critical clinical information, needed to make lifesaving decisions, not being available when those choices are being made. When trying to diagnose speed issues, the symptoms can be almost anywhere; the data network is much like the human central nervous system. Below is an overview of some of the places where problems may be found:

Part 1: The Cabling

Even wireless requires cabling to the wireless access points, but most commonly, cabling or fiber optic connections are provided to the desktop PC. Why is this a risk? Cabling can get wet and still function, but over time corrosion will occur, decreasing its reliability. During my first days at the HMO, a pipe burst (this happens in lots of hospitals) and flooded the cabling closet in the building. The cabling network provided a perfect path for the distribution of all of the water and it got into the cable that was only serving the phones at that point in time. The damaged cable had to be replaced so that calls could be completed without static on the line. Had we left it in place, it would have corroded to the point of being unusable.

Cabling can be inadvertently damaged or disconnected in the ceiling or floor by workers doing other work. Remember, the cable that is used for the computer often runs parallel to air conditioning ducts, plumbing, and cable TV wiring. I vividly remember receiving a call that our CEO's wireless access was not working in his office and I must correct the situation immediately. IT dispatched a technician to investigate and he found that the cable was disconnected in the ceiling. Upon further investigation, we found that the vendor for the security system (doors, cameras, etc.) had appropriated the cable for their own use because they could see that it didn't go all the way to a computer. They assumed it wasn't in use.

Many hospital organizations have a decentralized approach to cabling—the contractor for a remodeling job may install cable, a vendor will install the TV system, the security system, and the phone system, while the data network team and an electrician may install even more cables throughout the hospital. This decentralized approach occurs with increasing frequency because it's not glamorous technology. It's a challenging and dirty job that is often treated as a low funding priority in medical centers that don't step up and take responsibility. When the distribution infrastructure is shared, as is often unavoidable for cost containment reasons, there is always a risk that the connectivity provided via this cable will be disrupted. The other challenge is that even within IT, this role is often given a low level of importance. The cabling infrastructure is one of the most often overlooked elements in the building of a high-performing IT network, because it isn't visible.

Part 2: The Power

Electrical power is a primary thought in the planning of a hospital. Generators are used to provide emergency power should commercial power not be available. Many computers provide additional protection in the form of a small uninterruptible power source (UPS). The UPS systems typically have a very brief utilization cycle—five to fifteen minutes. Hospitals do an outstanding job planning for emergencies in these visible areas, but what about the areas that are not seen? When an architect is hired to design (or redesign) space, and when budget becomes a concern, the first place they look for "value engineering" is in the invisible areas.

Many hospitals have generators that will provide some electrical coverage in the event of a power failure, but the steps needed to provide total power to all outlets throughout the building is often not economically viable. However, when the delivery of clinical care to patients is dependent upon information on computers, all of the clinical computers must be connected to the generator power immediately. If any of the components described in this chapter are not on a continuous power supply, information may be lost or at a minimum not available when your physician is making lifesaving decisions.

Part 3: Environment Control

In 1998, I worked on a project that involved building a number of data center facilities in an existing medical center. It was a challenge just to get the space. When we began the design of the space, a consultant with whom I worked presented the case for a redundant air conditioning unit, indicating a belief that our aging chilled water air conditioning could easily compromise the viability of the systems we were installing. There were those who insisted that this was ridiculous because the medical center's chilled water-cooling system was sufficient, if untested, when required to sustain appropriate data center temperatures in the locations selected. Much of the success I've experienced in my career was built upon the knowledge and experience of working with this consultant who believed that technology infrastructure should be placed in an environment that was built using the "belt and suspenders" approach.

I supported the redundant choice and we proceeded, although it was at an additional cost. During the course of the project, an issue arose in the medical center and it was uncovered that the chilled water system was aging and unable to perform as needed. We were fortunate that our only decision was to use our redundant AC unit as primary, with a backup to the chilled water system. In data centers, the equipment will generate a good deal of heat. It is important that the physical infrastructure be designed to support whatever risks may occur. Another factor is that electronic records are more sensitive to water than paper is. Plan accordingly. In buildings that are more than five or ten years old, the air conditioning, plumbing, and electrical infrastructure may be the last to be updated; yet they are a primary requirement to access electronic medical information. These types of systems may not be updated until the facility moves into a new building.

Part 4: The Data Switch.

The data switch is a device that is used to connect multiple computers, wireless access points, or (in the case of Voice over IP) the phones to the network. It is plugged into the wall and it connects to the receiving devices via the cabling in the walls. Switches generally have a 100-meter (approximately 300 feet) limitation from the end device that they serve and are connected to the router using fiber optic cabling. The switch is designed to optimize the way information is transferred between locations. It provides a predefined amount of bandwidth to transmit data and when that predetermined limit is reached, information is still sent, but at a slower pace. The best example of this is e-mail. I'm sure you've noticed that if someone sends you an e-mail with a lot of information attached, it is frequently slower or takes longer to display. The interesting problem that occurs in data networks is that regardless of how much bandwidth you have, the information being sent will inevitably use it all—sometimes with good results, sometimes to the end user's frustration.

Part 5: The Router

The router is essentially a switch (see above) for switches. What this means is that multiple switches are connected back to a router that has even greater bandwidth capacity. The router then prepares the information and sends it to wherever the clinical information is stored. If the information is stored in another location, then one router sends the information to the distant router (there may be multiple routers in between, depending upon the distance being traveled and the network design). At that point, the router will send the information to a server that houses the application.

Part 6: The Server

This is where the application resides. It contains all of the rules for access, all of the data collected, all of the guidelines for identifying types of information, and the core application that follows the rules established when the application is designed. Some of these are off-the-shelf applications where the rules are highly standardized; some are customized by the customer to meet specific business requirements. All of the variable information is stored in the server. An example of this is the case of an organization that decided to install a Computerized Physician Order Entry (CPOE) system. One physician became very upset when entering a prescription for a patient and was quite vocal in his disapproval of the system. After he calmed down, a nurse with whom he had worked for many years pulled him aside and told him that he had been putting the decimal point in the wrong place on his prescriptions for years and the nursing staff had been correcting it for him. This type of human intervention will not happen in a CPOE, at least not yet. A server is programmed to behave in certain, specific ways, it will not make judgment calls, and it will not vary its approach, unless it is programmed to do so.

There are those who believe that the server is the most important part of the electronic information used in patient care. However, if any of the other parts fail to work, the server is little more than a paperweight, if you can find paper to hold down.

Part 7: The Storage

Most organizations have invested in electronic storage devices that contain all of the information collected over time. This information may appear to be innocuous at first, but if the storage systems fail, the computer-addressing methods may be unavailable, causing a major computer network outage where the computers needed for patient care cannot be accessed. If the entire record is only stored electronically, this can result in decisions being made with partial or incomplete information.

Chapter 8

Medical Records

In a perfect world, patients would walk into their physicians' offices, where they have an ongoing relationship and their medical history would be readily available. If you had to go to the hospital, your physician would be there waiting for you and would be the only person treating you. When you arrive at the hospital, you may not be conscious, you may have been in an accident, or you may be incoherent. You may be in shock from the event that brings you there. Imagine if these scenarios occurred when your physician is on vacation, at a seminar or treating another patient, or you are seen by someone who has none of the information listed in this paragraph?

When the information needed to treat you isn't readily available, the physician or nurse will try to complete a medical history, if you can speak. If you can't speak, they will ask anyone who may have accompanied you to the hospital for details and any related medical history. If there is no one to provide this information, they have to run tests and/or make educated guesses, depending upon the nature of your condition. They will go to your medical record to find out information needed to treat you, if they have it available.

The availability of your medical record is dependent upon these records being identified correctly. If you were previously admitted and the spelling of your name was off by one character or if the registration clerk spells your name wrong this time, they may find that no medical record exists and create another medical record. This means that the information from your past visit, the history, physical, lab results, chronic conditions—all of the previous information—may not be readily available to the treating physician. To illustrate this, please read the following:

Furley Lumpkin
Lee Lumpkin
Furly Lumpkin
Farley Lumpkin
Farly Lumpkin
F. Lee Lumpkin
Butch Lumpkin

These are obvious variations of the author's name; some are incorrect, but four of them are correct. They are all variations that I've seen on things from credit cards to transcripts. If a data entry or typographical error was made while entering your name, your record may not be found. It may depend upon whether the registration uses multiple forms of verification and if the staff takes the time to research the various options. If a department is really busy due to employee reductions or if it is late at night when staffing is already at a minimum threshold, your record may not be found.

The importance of your existing medical records, detailing any chronic conditions, medications, or allergies, cannot be overstated, especially if you are in a situation where you are unable to speak for yourself. This record can be used to determine what next steps need to be taken, what needs to be avoided, and whom to contact in the event of an emergency. It provides the physician with a frame of reference for who you are and what you may need. How do these doctors and nurses capture the information that they need in order to treat you, to avoid drug-drug interactions, to respond to the real issue versus one that has been there a long time, especially if it isn't related to why you are there today? They rely upon the medical record, if they can find it. If it is electronic, they have the identifying information to locate the electronic file, and the system is working, then they can gather all that they need.

Electronic Medical Record

The Electronic Medical Record (EMR) is a beginning, but it isn't a panacea. Anyone that has any experience with computers has experienced going to a Web site and trying to navigate to different places where information is supposed to be accessible, only to give up in frustration. There is the risk of information being "out of sight, out of mind," resulting in decisions that are made without medically necessary information. A mistake when buying something on-line has different ramifications than a mistake when treating a critically ill patient.

The concept of navigating through a variety of pages on a Web site or an application on a desktop computer is not intuitive to everyone in healthcare or any other field. Most people have had the experience of looking on a computer for information that was available, but couldn't be found because a space was missing or the alpha characters were case sensitive. There is a strong business case for using an EMR—and the rapid development and deployment of this technology is important to the future of healthcare—but we need to realistically understand that the costs and/or risks it may eliminate will be replaced by a new set of issues encountered by those using and supporting the system. The very traits that make a person an excellent caregiver may not match well with technology that isn't familiar to them. The human element in the implementation of these types of systems must be considered and tested with a standard protocol. Healthcare organizations must also be prepared to accommodate the additional training needed. Technology firms must commit to the development of tools that are intuitive to non-technical personnel.

If the EMR resides in the hospital, at one of your doctors' office, or at another hospital where you were treated, it may not be readily accessible in a crisis situation. Doctors and hospitals across the country have adopted different software applications, they use different medical record numbers, and you may have many different medical record numbers in one institution. The absence of standards for storing and sharing this information must be corrected in the short term for the systems to achieve their full potential. Creation of these standards is a step that very likely requires legislative action.

Ultimately, the best tool from a patient's perspective is one that can be utilized regardless of where you are seeking treatment and which is designed in such a way that the information is very secure, but accessible by medical professionals anytime you are admitted. The record needs to be application neutral. Imagine going into a hospital and someone telling you that they can't read your record because it is on the wrong type of paper. That is the metaphorical equivalent to incompatible computer applications and it is highly actionable. This is one of the three key challenges of this book: (1) for software manufacturers to place the needs of patients above the bottom line; (2) for legislators to take away accreditation status or funding if electronic medical records aren't implemented; and (3) for the consumers to insist on this standard availability. You rarely know ahead of time when you will need it.

The uses for portable information is significant—from the battlefield medic treating wounded soldiers and civilians, to the accident victim on vacation away from home, to the expectant mother bringing a life into the world a little early, or to the Emergency Medical Technician in an ambulance transporting a stroke or heart attack victim. Medical information provided quickly and easily so that it is readable by medical personnel can mean the difference between life and death.

There are communities that are looking into a portable medical record that can be accessed at any point of care under the auspices of the Regional Health Information Office (RHIO), regardless of the point of origin. However, the urgency to establish national standards is not widely understood, often leaving this off the table in political discussions.

CHAPTER 9

ELECTRICAL POWER: PLUGGING IN

Have you ever watched a scary movie where the setting was a vacant hospital? Did you wonder why it seemed creepy? Besides the absence of other people, it is the absence of light and power, two things taken for granted until they fail. It seems that most of the equipment in the hospital uses electrical power. The importance of this is sufficient to warrant designing a power plant that includes generators to provide electrical capacity to critical areas. The generators may have the ability to run the functions of the hospital from two hours to two weeks, depending upon the design and investment. Every individual part of a hospital's information or communication system requires power to operate, and when that power is not available, the information is not available.

In an emergency situation a generator will generally begin to function when there is a loss of commercial power to the building. This can be a complete loss or a partial loss, such as a brownout. When this loss or reduction in power occurs, there is a small window of time when the hospital may be completely without power, followed by a return with partial power. Some hospitals have invested in their generator capacity and electrical wiring to allow the generator to service the full operations of the hospital, but this requires a manual intervention in most cases and is only done when the outage is identified as sufficiently critical and long lasting enough to justify the utilization. During this window of time, there may be limited access to electronic information used in delivering your care, and some systems or applications may go into failure mode, requiring the intervention of the medical staff on duty.

Have you ever experienced a brief power outage at home? What happens to everything you have that is electrically powered, such as a cable box, the clock on your DVD player, the clock on your microwave? Do you have to go around resetting all of your clocks? Does your computer reboot? All of this happens. In a hospital setting, they may have their computers installed with a small uninterruptible power system (UPS) that bridges the gap between commercial and generator power for a few minutes. These are relatively inexpensive devices and well worth the investment on every computer in the hospital as we migrate to having more and more of our clinical planning on computers.

Telephone systems in hospitals are frequently designed to be powered through a much longer outage using UPS to avoid any risk of downtime and because the phone system is considered a life safety system. The time has come for the data network and infrastructure to be placed in this category, if it has not. Since both the voice and data networks are life safety systems, we should consider where they are placed.

When an architect looks at a building or design opportunity, obviously they want to create something of lasting function, originality, and beauty. They also want to create an environment of healing, with public areas that are serene and peaceful where patients and families can walk and refresh their mind, spirit, and heart. This is quite challenging to achieve, although many hotels do a phenomenal job of creating this type of indoor environment.

To create this environment, the data center or the telephone system is frequently placed below grade in a windowless area that may be at greater risk of flooding. In the 1970s, the Houston Medical Center area was hit by several large rainstorms that flooded the basements of these organizations. At that point, the data network was far less intricate and the phone system was not owned by the hospital, so the urgency in moving above grade wasn't there. Following the aftermath of Hurricane Katrina and Hurricane Rita, along with a number of other tropical storms/hurricanes, the urgency of moving these areas to a level that was above the flood plain greatly increased and many hospitals have begun to address this while remodeling or constructing new buildings. Architects and contractors need to know that an eight-inch water pipe that bursts in the data center or on the telephone system has an organizational impact that could be every bit as severe as a hurricane, a tornado, an earthquake, power loss due to wildfires, or other disaster, regardless of the source.

A normal commercial building will spend 30 percent of their total operating expense on energy. This is per Energy Star, a joint program of the U.S. Environmental Protection Agency and the U.S. Department of Energy. While the percentage of the total operating budget is smaller in a hospital, it is an exceptionally important line item on the budget and is a major part of the hospital's overhead costs. Beyond the cost factor, the hospital needs to look at long-term sustainability, should the power grid be compromised for any reason. In the aftermath of the Northridge earthquake of 1994 in California, laws were passed that required hospitals around the state to be retrofitted to withstand an earthquake of significant magnitude. The requirements did not stipulate that these hospitals be built beyond "code" to incorporate alternative power sources that are not included in the various current building codes. However, given the criticality of continuous power to the hospital environment, hospitals should be designed to include alternative energy sources.

If a hospital were to move completely off of the power grid by harnessing wind power or solar power, the savings in cost could have a material impact on the cost of healthcare in the United States. At a minimum this would mitigate the risk of brownouts and power failures on sensitive, life-safety systems that are happening with increasing frequency due to the increased demand and our aging infrastructure. Hospitals should be conducting comprehensive audits of their energy performance and identifying a ten-year plan to help them become certified for Leadership in Energy and Environmental Design (LEED). According to the April, 2008, issue of *Tierra Grande, Journal of the Real Estate Center at Texas A&M University*, "the LEED system has become the nationally accepted benchmark for design, construction and operation of high performance green buildings." Ideally, the hospital would endeavor for the platinum certification, but whatever level it strives to achieve should be a factor in the overall survey of the hospital. Is it ridiculous to ask if your hospital is a "green building?"

The undertaking to migrate to alternative fuel sources, such as harnessing wind and solar power, is a monumental change that may be driven by the ever-increasing power demands of the hospital's technology infrastructure. Regardless of your belief about global warming, it is irresponsible for a healthcare organization to continue to demand more and more power without looking at what can be done to reduce their demand on the power grid. This issue is a growing one in our communities—and shouldn't our community-based hospitals be leaders and innovators in this endeavor?

Chapter 10

Telecommunications

One area where technology is driving rapid change is voice telecommunications. You may have heard of Voice over IP and thought, "Big deal, this doesn't apply to me." However, telecommunications manufacturers are forcing this to apply to you. Without going into too much detail, Voice over Internet Protocol (VoIP) is the use of the data network to transmit voice calls. This is highly efficient, but is dependent upon the reliability of the data network. The viability of this is best determined by asking yourself if you know the number for telephone repair or if the computer help desk number is more widely known.

Regardless of your point of view, IP is the primary focus for development of new systems in the voice telecommunications field. This becomes vital in designing the voice network and setting expectations correctly because as long as the networks are separate, when one fails, there is another way to communicate to the outside world, whether that world is down the hall, in another building, or in a central monitoring station.

This isn't the first time a technological shift has driven major changes in the telecommunications arena. There have been incremental changes over the last 100+ years, such as when Touch-Tone replaced dial phones or when the ability to dial long distance was introduced in the late 1950s. This is the first major technological shift since the divestiture of AT&T and the Regional Bell Operating Companies and is being done without significant regulation. Why is this important to you as a hospital patient? If you are a patient and you need nursing assistance, you may press a nurse call button and if that doesn't work, you might call the hospital operator. Interestingly, in even our most fragile state, many people can think to dial zero for operator, when all else fails. In a converged network transporting telephone calls and electronic data over a common network, when one fails, they all fail. Imagine the impact of placing all of our systems on one network and the risk to patients in the hospital. Imagine this scenario in a Katrina-type event or a terrorist attack.

Due to the design of IP infrastructure, there are distance limitations between the end device and the network equipment. These limitations are not the same as what is required on the phone network, where a phone may be several thousand feet away from the main telephone system. This begs the question, why can't the two co-exist on the same network? They can, but when doing so, the network must be designed with an understanding of the impact single points of failure can have in a hospital environment. Accreditation bodies should require that all hospitals using Voice over IP clearly have a medical grade network that is very fault tolerant and highly redundant, and it should be validated as part of the survey, something that is most likely going to be driven by the clinical information used on the data network rather than an understanding of the importance of the telephone network.

Locating a Patient in a Disaster

Under federal HIPAA guidelines as they are interpreted today, if you call to locate a family member you may not find them for a lot of reasons. If you are in the emergency room, you may not be a registered patient, so the hospital operator may have no idea who you are or where you are. If you are in the waiting room of the emergency room waiting to be seen, fewer records may exist. If the call is routed to the right area, where you are waiting or being treated and they ask for "Betty," but your registration is under "Elizabeth," the caller will be out of luck. The short answer to this situation is that your friends and family need to be prepared to ask for you by your given name.

Locating a family member at a hospital in a major metropolitan area can be difficult when you don't know where they've been taken. In a horrific event, such as September 11th, where the casualties may be quite high, the problem is magnified and it is an element of planning for disasters, which has been largely overlooked. Perhaps a patient information clearinghouse could be established and activated in a disaster and publicized. Perhaps a number like 311, which is for non-emergent calls to the police and fire.

One of the major issues in New York City immediately following September 11, 2001, was that people thought the phones didn't work. Technically most phones were still working, but due to the overload of callers, the network was slow to respond and it could take minutes to get a dial tone on a landline. These callers quickly focused on the New York City hospitals trying to locate missing loved ones, co-workers, neighbors, and friends. This call volume then caused the ripple effect of causing the phone systems in the hospitals to appear unworkable, making the ability to communicate around the medical centers a greater challenge than normal.

Emergency Number Standardization

Another important opportunity for improvement via standardization in hospitals is the numbering plan for internal calls. These codes will likely vary from hospital to hospital, even if the same umbrella corporation owns them. These codes may be anywhere from one to five digits depending upon how the system is designed. Due to staff shortages in nursing around the country, many nurses may work at several different hospitals over the course of the year. Their jobs would be made easier if the number for calling security or a code blue was standardized, much like 911, 411, or 311 are today. The value to patients and staff is obvious. This would be a minor change in most phone systems.

Making Telephone Calls in the Hospital

Some of you may not remember, but there was a time when telephone calls didn't come in "buckets of minutes" or on "calling plans"; they were charged incrementally. The first three minutes and then each additional minute was called "overtime" and was priced well above the $.01-04 per minute we see today. As "the phone company" was opened to competition these charges began to decrease for a wide variety of reasons. This savings has not been passed on to many hospital patients for some very interesting reasons that are worth a little exploration.

Hospitals, health systems, and hotels subscribe to lines that are provided by various carriers, just like most of us do. However, they have an extra advantage—these carriers know that they have a captive audience for their services and as a result, they offer financial incentives in the form of commission checks that are used to offset the cost of telephone calls in the hospital. Payphones, such as those in waiting areas, also generate commissions.

These special lines are usually set up to be accessed by patients only and require the caller to use a credit card or other billing method. When placing a call the carrier adds a surcharge on to the price of the call to make their profit and to pay the hospital or hotel their commission. The amount of the surcharge is determined by the amount of commission the hospital wants to receive. These revenues are then used to calculate the total income for the hospital.

While that seems to be reasonable, unlike hotels, many hospitals have taken the additional step of banning the use of cell phones in all areas of the hospital, citing concerns about interference. Cellular interference with medical equipment is a topic of importance and to understand the issue, you need to understand the source of the interference. A cell phone continuously sends very low-level signals to the cellular network so that when a call is placed to the subscriber, the cellular network knows where to send the call. This signal increases when the device is activated to receive a call or to place a call. This is why the battery goes dead even when you don't use the phone. Older model cell phones had to put out a much stronger signal to stay connected to the network. The newer models (since 2000) have continued to lower the power output. To our knowledge, there have been no incidents of verifiable failure of medical equipment due to the use of cell phones. If the interference were an issue, the use of wireless computers in a medical center would also be suspect.

Due to the "cell phone ban," the patient, who is lying in the bed with nothing but a hospital gown on, has to have the presence of mind to remember a credit card number on which to charge the call. Of course, they could leave their credit card lying out on the bedside table, risking the loss or theft of the card. Additionally, hospitals are driving the less acutely sick patients out of the hospital into ambulatory settings, so if you are unfortunate enough to be sufficiently ill to be hospitalized with bills in the thousands of dollars, why doesn't the hospital let you make calls throughout a reasonable local calling area? It's just business.

Having worked in two major hospitals in a decision-making role, I made the choice that we would allow our patients free calling in the five surrounding area codes. The sky didn't fall; in fact, I continued to keep this cost-effective by pushing our vendors for lower contract calling rates. The budgetary impact on the hospital was not noticeable. We didn't advertise it, we just told people how to call, and when they needed to call their family and loved ones, they did, without breaking their bank or ours. We even expanded this to house phones in the main hospital so that physicians could call their answering service or office without incurring these charges. That was a big win with the physicians. Again, no bank was broken.

I would like to tell you that I made this decision from a completely altruistic point of view, but unfortunately I made it after learning of an horrific experience a patient had in one of my hospitals. The patient was a middle-aged, homeless man, with no means of paying for calls. He'd been estranged from his family for a long time and had just been told that his condition was terminal, with the time he had left calculated in hours. He called the hospital operator to make the call and she refused because he had no means of paying for it. She was doing her job to the best of her ability and she knew that cost containment was a big issue for the hospital. Her actions changed hospital policy for thousands of patient stays in the coming years. Unfortunately, he died without ever making contact with his family.

Chapter 11

Non-IT Systems

The use of Internet Protocol (IP) is now integral to most systems used in a hospital in one way or another and the speed of implementation has been faster—more than any hospital could possibly keep up with. One reason is that it may appear to be an inexpensive tool for monitoring or accessing a system. This rapid growth has forced the evolution of jobs from various backgrounds into that of "specialists" that operate under the radar of IT and who have learned how to ask for connection to the hospital data network without clearly identifying or understanding the risk imposed by this access. These roles are necessary, and in order to be successful, every IT organization has to acknowledge their existence and work with them to ensure their needs are understood. Reporting structures for these roles are unimportant when IT has a strong, mutually respectful relationship with colleagues in other departments.

The IT Department has historically viewed "Job One" as network security, not policing how it is used. Only as the use has become more pervasive and issues more intrusive have they begun to get interested in these more remote systems/applications, such as nurse call, infusion pumps, cardiac monitors, etc. These systems may be applications that are unique to a department and which are running on a PC that someone set up to track research results or data.

Most hospitals are conducting security audits and deal with the issues as they appear in the subsequent report on the security of the hospital network. What many haven't done is a comprehensive assessment of all areas to determine what happens operationally if a part or the entire network fails.

Many leaders in healthcare IT Departments are technologists first and lack the skills needed to deal effectively with quasi-technical or non-technical personnel. There is sometimes a bit of an elitist atmosphere that supposes that anyone who doesn't understand technology isn't "smart" or at most is not as smart as they are. This attitude creates the single greatest risk of failure in any technology organization. Two types of people will populate a strong, high performing IT organization: (1) those that are strong technologists and (2) those that are out in front of the changes, helping translate issues and expectations back and forth between the end user and the technologist.

Technology can make major changes in our medical system, but it will also introduce new areas of risks that are not going to be realized until there are catastrophic outages. These outages will be the topic of peer-to-peer reviews, protected by attorney/client privilege, and attended by risk management, all of which are appropriate. It is extraordinarily unlikely that you will ever know such an event occurred, and how, why, or what steps are being taken to prevent it from happening again.

Another essential function of an IT leader is to ensure that value is being added when capital investments and operational changes are occurring. Cost increases in healthcare are significantly driven by what IT needs to spend. As anyone who has owned a PC knows, there is a constant need to upgrade hardware or software because a vendor determines that enough changes have been made to warrant a new version. Another cost that is sometimes overlooked is the annual licensing fees required to ensure ongoing support. Many vendors will refuse to provide support if you haven't paid your annual licensing fee or if you are not running a current version of software on current hardware.

This is their right in a free market, but the downside is the ever increasing and unsustainable cost of healthcare. What is missing in the equation is the social conscience and motivation needed to force manufacturer's to stop creating content neutral upgrades. There is no doubt that periodic upgrades are important, but having applications that are backwards and forwards compatible isn't impossible, if we have the will to do so. Product life cycle management for major IT costs needs to be a primary role of the IT leadership. They need to be communicating back to the vendors that these predatory content neutral upgrades are driving the costs of healthcare beyond a level that can be sustained. We spend money lobbying Congress to pass various healthcare bills, but don't take the same initiative when addressing one of our fastest growing line items of cost in healthcare.

Businesses that are open 24/7 often have a reduced staff in the all-night shift. Part of what makes that feasible is that the functions needed within the in-patient areas are reduced due to lower volume. Perhaps they decided that they could monitor cardiac patients from a centralized location using IP. If they make this choice, it is essential that they have instant communication with the staff remaining on the floor so that they can respond if your alarms aren't heard.

There are many non-IT type systems that are now moving towards using IP protocol. Departments such as bio-medical engineering or facilities management often appropriately manage these systems because someone in those departments who has learned about network equipment in any combination of ways has requested that they be provided an IP address. The IT Department does not know how/why this is being used and as such, rarely has an accurate assessment of whether or not the system is mission critical, life-safety, or incidental. When network or application upgrades occur, there may be a "planned down," which means there is a predetermined period of time when the network or application will be off-line, making it inaccessible.

Large software companies don't make all of their money selling new software, they also make it by selling upgrades to applications. These upgrades occur with increasing frequency and have life cycles that are unacceptably short. Unfortunately, hospitals and IT organizations within hospitals often fail to take the initiative to confront the application developers, or the software and hardware vendors. Many healthcare IT people came from this industry or aspire to work in that field, so they don't want to risk making enemies when pointing out the issue. The net result is that they accept a vendor telling them their software or hardware is approaching "end of life" and will no longer be supported. The business case that existed to justify some technological changes is often reduction in staff hours, but the annual maintenance, license fees, and upgrade costs rapidly eat away at these perceived values, and few institutions follow through on evaluating a business case in the information technology arena because they don't understand the issues.

Chapter 12

Enter with Caution

When you enter a hospital, you are entering a world that is very different from the one you experience on a day-to-day basis. In many situations you would rather not be there, but have no choice if you want to live. The hospital will do everything they can to soothe your worries and many of the medical professionals you will encounter are among the most dedicated and compassionate people you will ever meet. However, "the hospital" is a business. They have a motto, a slogan, a mission, a vision statement, or all of these; however, words are meaningless if they do not operationalize their motto/slogan/mission/vision into their everyday work life. To paraphrase a popular advertising slogan, what happens in the hospital, stays in the hospital, would more likely be the truth behind the motto/slogan/mission/vision. There are things you need to know about what is happening while you are in the hospital, what is being done to you and for you. You should never be hesitant to ask.

We each have the personal obligation to equip ourselves with an understanding of the environment when life throws challenges at us, regardless of their source. "Don't bother the doctors." "Leave the nurses alone." I remember my mother telling me this when my father had his first heart attack. I was living 200 miles away and couldn't get there to find out what was going on. Prior to this, my knowledge of the healthcare system in the U.S. was limited mostly to third party stories, the occasional newspaper article, or the horror story of someone who won a malpractice lawsuit. The only person I knew that was a party to a malpractice lawsuit was my cousin's mother-in-law, who smelled alcohol on the breath of her doctor just before her surgery. She tried unsuccessfully to stop them from putting her under. During the surgery, the doctor made a serious mistake, disabling her for life.

The practice of medicine and providing care to people in need strikes an altruistic chord in most people. It is the bridge from life to death that fascinates and horrifies us. My journey toward a career in healthcare began by working for Southwestern Bell and ultimately AT&T, when it was known simply as "the telephone company." They offered a unique educational experience that was instrumental in leading me to work in the healthcare field, first for a large health maintenance organization (HMO) and then for a major metropolitan hospital in Los Angeles. During my years in healthcare, I had the great fortune of working with many very dedicated people who shared my sense of purpose and who have devoted their entire lives to this effort. If you have access and a means to pay for it, the United States has the best health system in the world. Our challenge continues to be finding new, better ways to provide universal access to healthcare.

After leaving my most recent position in healthcare at a major medical center on the West Coast, I kept encountering story after story that echoed what I had seen from the inside and as a family member assisting relatives and friends in the hospitals in other parts of the country when they were ill. Sitting in restaurants, people told me their stories. Flying to visit my family became an insightful experience when the person seated next to me found out about my work. There were stories of healthcare issues everywhere I turned. If there was ever any doubt in my mind, a friend called one day to discuss the concept of a book he was thinking about that mirrored what I had already begun and we began our collaboration on this book.

When I left the West Coast hospital, I wanted to write about some of the things I had learned in my nearly twenty years in healthcare. Shortly before I began making notes for this book, I saw the movie *Sicko* by Michael Moore, and soon thereafter, I read the front-page *Los Angeles Times* story on July 15, 2007, titled "Footnotes to a Tragedy." Within days, I read the July 23, 2007, issue of *People* magazine article titled "Coverage Denied" that prompted me to provide my insight into the world of healthcare.

During the writing of this book, a highly publicized case of medication error involving the infant children of actor Dennis Quaid occurred. His infant twins were administered a potentially fatal dose of medicine in error. His subsequent testimony before Congress in May, 2008, also served to influence this book. He explained that he believed that our society is sometimes overly litigious, but through the experience with his children, he learned that sometimes the only way to achieve sustainable change is to force it legally.

The topic of avoidable errors continues to be headline news, with Lindsey Tanner of the Associated Press reporting on April

7, 2008, "Drug errors affect one in fourteen children." Dr. Charles Homer of the National Initiative conducted the study she is quoting for Children's Healthcare Quality. This analysis was only on pediatric cases; imagine the rate in adult cases.

Recently my older brother had surgery and experienced a number of complications, including medication errors. Following the second of a two-stage surgical procedure, he experienced numerous problems. When having a post-operative consultation, the first question the doctor asked was, "Has he had a stroke?" This sent us into panic mode. Our frame of reference for him was as a healthy sixty-four-year-old with chronic back problems, but no other noticeable issues. The physician asking the question was a neurologist whose only frame of reference was the man lying in the bed in front of her who looked older than his years and who clearly had experienced some sort of traumatic event. Then she told us that he had Bells Palsy, which was treatable using medication that was contraindicated following the type of surgery he had.

When he was transferred to the rehab facility, I continued to protest that something else was wrong because even the neurologist acknowledged that she had never seen a case of Bells Palsy as a result of this type of surgery. The treating physician in rehab would not question the previous doctor's orders or diagnosis. Apparently his rehab physician concluded we were right, although he never said so. He stopped treating Bells Palsy, there was immediate improvement, and my brother was home within a week. I am convinced that the outcome would have been very different if we hadn't politely protested and allowed the rehab physician to raise questions of his own behind the scenes. We were never told what happened and were satisfied that he was getting better quickly with the medication change. Doctors and nurses do their best, but their frame of reference for how patients appear and act is very limited, especially during some of the worst moments of a patient's life. How we appear and what we can and cannot do are part of the equation when evaluating our condition. If you cannot speak for yourself, it is important to have people who can speak for you, with knowledge of your life and abilities.

Chapter 13

Who are the employees of a hospital?

The staff in the hospital are people, like us. They have good days and bad. Sometimes they come to work worried about their finances, their love life (or lack thereof), the rebellion of a teenage child, a cheating spouse, or a sick relative across the country. They have the same problems and frailties that we do. Some are alcoholics, some are drug addicts, and some are in denial of their condition or the impact it has on their judgment. Some are control freaks; some micromanagers, and some have no bedside manner. These are the everyday, ordinary people who do the extraordinary—they give hope. It is imperative that we overlay any understanding of the healthcare field with this understanding of our shared humanity.

Nurses have a designated work schedule, just like many other professions. The difference is that there must be someone continuously available to take on the role of the nurse as shifts change. Just like the rest of us, a nurse may get ill on their way to work and report out at the last minute, they may have car trouble, childcare issues, or other situations that prevent them from being there for their assigned shift. Finding a replacement person to cover the shift isn't easy. To do this, an administrator has to balance the number of hours a nurse has already worked in the preceding twenty-four hours, evaluate the staffing ratio required based upon the criticality of the patient, then find someone who is available and can get there in a reasonable time frame. Given the shortage of nurses, this is a far more difficult task than one might think.

The nurse that is asked to fill the vacated shift must meet licensing requirements, have completed basic life support (BLS) training, as well as a number of other specialty-related training modules. In addition to this, they are accountable for adherence to the hospital's policies and procedures. In the absence of a nurse with this knowledge, the hospital may select a registry nurse who has worked at three or four hospitals in the past week, each with their own set of policies and procedures. It is up to that nurse to remember which is which because they vary from hospital to hospital.

Hospitals are required to have detailed policies and procedures (P&Ps) describing the actions to be taken in various relatively common administrative and clinical situations. These used to be kept in binders located at each nursing station and in each department. More often than not, these are now on an internal Web site and annual reviews of all P&Ps are not consistently enforced and documented. So why do hospitals have them at all? Protection when something goes wrong.

Greater than having the time or taking the time to read hospital P&Ps, is the challenge of managing the information they describe. Hospital policies and procedures are not or should not be confidential and should be accessible by any patient or interested community member. In a large hospital, if anyone goes to the Web to search for a particular topic in the hospital P&Ps, you may get multiple P&Ps on the same topic, but each may have been written without the awareness of the others, requiring a major coordination effort should changes be made in one that affects the others. Alternatively, your end product may be inherently conflicting instructions. There may be a complete lack of standardization. Surveyors should consider going to a computer to browse various topics such as any of the hospital's code names.

Annual staff testing for knowledge of these policies and procedures should be put in place and documented for review by hospital leadership and accreditation agencies. It might seem that clinical policies would only come from clinical areas, but areas such as bio-medical engineering, the TV shop, the IT department, and Telecom may also have P&Ps that relate to clinical issues and procedures, which require testing.

An inherent flaw of technology is that you only see what you open. There may be twenty P&Ps on a certain topic, but you open the first one and your system has identified twenty possible options. If you read the first one and get the information you want or validate what you thought, you may choose to ignore additional information that has changed, but not been coordinated. There is no arbitrator to determine which policy is the most relevant to your situation other than you.

Searching for information may be a bit like searching for a needle in a haystack and since you can't see the haystack, you are at a loss as to where or how deep to look. You have no way of knowing if you've exhausted your options or not. The Web is a great tool. However, if hospitals are going to use this tool for P&P storage, then new methods for reviewing all of the posted P&Ps must be created to ensure that all staff knows and understands them. This understanding should be established by the leadership of the hospital, regardless of status, from MDs to consultants on site, from the environmental services staff to the CEO.

Technology can be adapted to validate and electronically document that every employee has read and been tested on the P&Ps that are relevant to their area. Hospitals must be held accountable for ensuring that their P&Ps are standardized or at least categorized in a uniform way so that staff can find information quickly. Equally important, as changes occur, there must be a secure, verifiable method of validating that the employee has read and understands the P&Ps. In the past this was done using an "in-service" signature sheet signed by all employees in a work area and the accrediting agency validated that employees, contractors, vendors, and volunteers had done this. Anyone who enters the hospital building(s) is a potential risk to a patient because of the germs they carry and should be required to know and follow these procedures.

A homeless patient is discharged from a hospital and dropped off on skid row in Los Angeles; a patient lies on the floor of an emergency room coughing up blood while the staff ignores them, mops the floor around them, and tells them to call 911; a patient is mugged within a few hundred feet of a hospital's emergency room doors; a patient dies while being driven around in an ambulance to multiple hospitals who have temporarily closed their emergency rooms due to exceeding their capacity; or a celebrity's children become the victims of a careless and easily avoidable medication error that was so common that the error type is categorized as "look alike/sound alike" errors—these are all things that have happened in hospitals of varying status levels, from among the best to hospitals that were subsequently closed.

The issue of look alike/sound alike medication is particularly disturbing because it isn't new and it continues because hospitals continue to allow the confusion to exist. Isn't this an effort worthy of the time of the hospital leadership in conjunction with organizations such as the various political action committees?

Should they only be lobbying Congress? Why not lobby the pharmaceutical companies? It would seem to be a good fit and they would carry a great deal of clout when representing their members. However, hospital leaders are often too focused on internal politics, their next career move, business cases, or revenue collection to remember that the #1 reason they exist is to care for their patients, whether they are an MD, an RN, a PA, or the janitor that is mopping the floor.

Reformative steps are not often taken until a problem sees the light of day— sometimes referred as the glare of the media spotlight. The issue has to grab headlines, a special on a news show, or be highlighted in a movie. Patient's fall victim to medication errors because drugs look and sound alike and are sometimes packaged alike. When administered there are very different outcomes—but this often doesn't become headline news until a celebrity has a personal experience with this and can force the issue through their own access to the media.

Our hospital leadership is failing in some cases by being too focused on problems that have nothing to do with patient care. The responsibility for the performance of a hospital rests squarely on the shoulders of the hospital leadership. They have the opportunity and the obligation to demand action, whether this action is directed at their own staff or from pharmaceutical companies. Hospital leaders are connected to organizations around the world that meet regularly to talk about a variety of issues and they have the opportunity to use their voice to completely eliminate issues such as look alike/sound alike medications.

Chapter 14

Not-For-Profit Hospitals

According to the Web site of the American Hospital Association, the total number of registered hospitals in the United States is 5,747, of which 4,297 are considered community hospitals. A community hospital is just what it sounds like—a hospital with the purpose of serving a specific community of interest. This may be geographic or religious. Not-for-profit and government-owned hospitals constitute 82 percent of the total. Community hospitals are responsible for 35,377,659 admissions per year, which is 95 percent of total annual admissions.

The different types of hospitals are partially determined by how they are incorporated and their filings with the IRS. Only 18% of the registered hospitals in the United States are for-profit. The for-profit hospitals are often a series of shell corporations that are designed to optimize the potential for profit for the owners or shareholders. For purposes of the examples used herein, we will focus on variations of the not-for-profit models.

To be a not-for-profit organization a company has to meet a number of criteria, beginning with a commitment to help a community of people with common interests. When they make money, they are required to reinvest any unused funds or income into capital expenditures in the following year. Their designation as a not-for-profit institution is a tax incentive for serving people from all walks of life, regardless of their ability to pay.

If a hospital or medical practice is a not-for-profit entity, receiving tax incentives from the American people, then why are they allowed to destroy the financial life of the patient or their family? Should a person be forced into bankruptcy or have their credit destroyed when they are unable to pay a hospital bill when the basis of the hospital's tax exempt status is their taking care of charitable cases? How do they define charitable cases? If someone needs medical attention and isn't able to pay for it, is that charity or a bad debt? It depends upon the accountant.

The flip side of the question then becomes how do we ensure the payment of medical expenses to organizations that receive tax benefits based on their acceptance of charitable cases, when in fact, this treatment is part of their mission driven by their not-for-profit status? One method might be to have the individual report any forgiven debt as part of their tax return and the cancellation of any tax refund that might be applicable to them for a period of time, without adding additional tax liabilities for the forgiven debt. At the same time, the not-for-profit organizations should be prevented from destroying a person's financial life when they've experienced a catastrophic illness.

Understanding this issue is complex and the not-for-profit status in healthcare needs closer examination. In the following you will find a couple of hospital business models that illustrate the need for change.

Example 1

As an example, "Big HMO" (Health Maintenance Organization) is a privately held company that owns a number of other affiliated businesses, including its own hospitals, as a separate line of business with their own unique tax ID. In one region the affiliated medical group is a partnership of physicians operating under the safety of the HMO's umbrella, and in another it is a corporation operating under that same umbrella. The corporate umbrella provides various economies of scale through centralized purchasing/acquisition of assets, staff resources, technology infrastructure, etc. Their hospitals are operated as a not-for-profit entity, while the remainder of their corporations and partnerships may or may not be part of a for-profit business model.

At Big HMO the hospitals provide a variety of services to the for-profit side of the business, but funds many of these costs in the not-for-profit (NFP) hospital budget. For example, their monthly telephone bill, electric bill, water, sewage, environmental staff, engineers, biomedical engineers, and on and on may be funded through the hospital. What this effectively does is to allow much of the cost of day-to-day medical group operational costs to be off-loaded to the NFP entity. Are the "for profit" entities owned by a not-for-profit organization being taxed on the benefits they receive from the not-for-profit entity?

If the NFP entity is receiving special tax consideration from any government organization, then they are accountable for their actions to you—the taxpayer. Equally important, they must be held accountable for their spending on projects that skyrocket out of control. It is their avoidance of profit through shell games such as we described above that places a greater tax burden on each of us. These costs are part of the financial infrastructure of the hospitals in big HMOs and are often incorporated into their pricing models, artificially driving up the cost of hospitalization in this country.

To guarantee success, many will hire consulting firms to advise them on business practices, to introduce new technology, and implement systems and applications. This has become a billion dollar industry. When the final work is completed, the consultant's advice may be completely ignored, but they will have received their payday and their point of view is frequently that it is ultimately "the business owner's decision" whether or not to implement their recommendations. Consultants have delivered the service for which their customer hired them, providing opinions, best practices, and professional guidance that is often overlooked or which is impractical in the operational reality of a hospital.

Large change efforts in an organization like a hospital or HMO can be very costly economically, but also from an internal political point of view. Consultants can come into an organization and push through change without much regard for the organization's culture or the long-term impact of their actions. Since change is often resisted, this needs to be very carefully and closely managed or the project staff can get out of control and out of touch with the very people who are supposed to utilize the new application or process.

Example 2

Another example is a giant monolithic building located in the center of town under a big sign that reads "Metropolitan Hospital" (MH). That is all one organization, isn't it? Let's say you are transported there by ambulance to their emergency room. Once you cross the threshold everything is labeled with the same logo, everything is clearly branded as MH. Everyone you encounter wears a badge that identifies him or her as employees of

MH. The reality will vary between locations, but it is entirely possible that MH has a contract with a medical group to operate the ER and that medical group is incorporated and may be for profit, operating behind the sign of MH. Many hospitals have difficulty finding physicians that will accept emergency room cases and they forego having privileges at a hospital rather than take on the financial burden of these uninsured patients. The only way around this is for the hospital to financially incentivize the physician or for practices to use the role of a "hospitalist." A hospitalist is a member of a physician practice or a contractor that handles hospital patients so that the other physicians are not encumbered with making rounds or treating less profitable cases. The hospitalist may be a requirement of the insurance plan or may be something that a private practice puts in place. Most importantly, the hospitalist often doesn't know you and you lose the personal touch that makes for the best outcome.

Now that you have been seen by the emergency room physician at Example 2 (MH), the physician may determine that you need an x-ray or an MRI. You are transported through the halls of MH to the Radiology Department, where you are met by more employees of MH. Again, this department may be a for-profit practice, making it completely separate from a billing standpoint. This is why you get so many different bills after one hospital stay.

You have had your x-ray or MRI and now are being admitted, but part of the admissions process is completing labs so that your medical team fully understands your condition. In comes a lab tech with a badge indicating that he or she is an employee of MH. The phlebotomist drawing your blood probably is an employee, but then takes your samples to a lab that may be an outsourced contract with a for profit corporation. Examples can go on and on.

Making a profit in the medical field is completely legitimate, but let's be straightforward so that a true understanding of the real costs of providing healthcare is clear. The tax credits that are given to NFPs are valuable incentives, but they are also a public trust. This is a trust that requires medical care beyond just stabilizing of the patient.

Chapter 15

Consultants in Not-For-Profit Hospitals

There is no greater risk of financial improprieties than in the engagement of consultant experts who are hired to make recommendations about actions they believe would be viable and to help the senior management identify the level of pain these changes will cause within their organization. Consulting practices can provide exceptional value to an organization, but only if they have specific identifiable and sustainable outcomes. These firms are used to provide information about "best practices" that are used in other hospitals, to provide recommendations for changes in processes within the hospital organization, and they may be engaged to analyze the economic viability of a line of business that the hospital is considering.

These firms rarely offer any guarantee of positive outcomes, improved patient care, or warranty for the accuracy of the recommendations they make. However, they often offer one thing—they drive up costs while disguising their efforts as cost-containment efforts and this impacts the cost of healthcare to everyone. The expenses are passed along through higher medical costs that are then forwarded along into higher health insurance premiums. These consultants will rarely be visible to you as a patient, but you should be aware that these people that may not have all of information needed and/or who have no accountability for their outcomes are shaping decisions made within the hospital.

Healthcare consulting is a cottage industry that has grown a into major business expenditure for some hospitals. These consulting firms are engaged to advise on financial processes, business processes, system selection, business cases, departmental organizational structure, and clinical best practices used at other hospitals. Consulting fees are a cost of doing business, are factored into the hospital budget, and are ultimately passed on to the public in the prices the hospitals charge.

Consulting is an industry with low accountability for outcomes and potentially a high profitability. The outcomes are completely dependent upon the work ethic, knowledge, and integrity of the major participants in the engagement. Many consulting arrangements are based upon a loosely worded letter of engagement, which may or may not include a number of key specific items, such as milestones for delivery of their service or any *verifiable*, proven track record of expertise.

Consultants typically charge for billable hours plus expenses. Most consultants are rarely locally based and travel to their consulting engagement site. They are supported by a network of staff in the headquarters that conducts research for them on subjects of interest or importance. They stay in hotels, order room service, drive rental cars, eat at nice restaurants, and even have their laundry done at the expense of the engaging organization. Their expenses are generally considered a normal cost of doing business, but the consulting firm then will add a "processing" fee of 10 to 15 percent for handling the expenses of the consultant. A small consulting engagement can easily be $500,000 and all of this may be incurred without a competitive bid or even proper oversight of the costs.

Consulting engagements in healthcare represent a significant risk for inappropriate selection based upon a consultant's unsubstantiated "expertise" in a given area. This expertise may or may not be translatable into value for the engaging organization. A consulting firm may be engaged to implement large-scale information technology or information systems projects, conduct a business process redesign, or improve the organization's cash flow. Every day hospital staff are being squeezed, forced to do more and more with less and less, yet the costs of healthcare continues to rise. Insurance companies are driving healthcare providers and hospitals to report performance and using this information to validate the cost/value relationship. Many hospitals are not consistently driving similar efforts with the consulting firms they use.

Hospitals should consider forcing pay for performance on all consulting firms they utilize. This can be changed if the consulting letter of engagement contains enforceable clauses for payment that are contingent upon achieving insights into the business operations of the hospital based upon the knowledge of their highly valued subject matter experts. The reality is that consultants often have subject matter expertise in theory only and have not been sufficiently successful in the marketplace to validate this expertise. If they have the expertise as they indicate, then taking a job on a contingency with progress payments based upon specific milestones should not be a significant risk factor to them.

Ultimately the outcome is the responsibility of the management and executive team of the hospital. Any hospital organization that engages a consulting firm and doesn't achieve verifiable, sustainable improvement, should consider the long-term viability of the hospital executive staff. This action alone would change the landscape of consulting firms that operate around healthcare organizations.

The challenge of holding executives accountable for the outcome is that they may choose to move to another, more lucrative opportunity before their outcomes are measured. In high-profile organizations, it is possible that executives join for the exclusive purpose of being able to take credit for making a major change and then leave before the change has been verified as successful. They may enter at a time when finances are plentiful and might never endure the economic and emotional aftermath of their actions during a reversal of fortunes. For this reason, it is imperative that accountability be established before, during, and after the completion of an initiative.

Avoiding these pitfalls is relatively simple, if every major initiative in a business has a strongly developed business case, including the engagement of consultants. A business case is developed by evaluating the impact a proposed change or action will have on the financial performance of the organization. These business cases are often very subjective and rarely does the executive leadership of the hospital require the project leaders to validate the achievement of the outcomes forecasted in their initial business case. The engagement of consulting firms should be specific, with a defined outcome and timeline. The use of consulting firms in healthcare should be far less commonplace. The business case may not improve cash flow, it may not reduce costs, but the forecasted outcome should always be known and it should be comprehensive.

Too often business cases are developed that overlook key ingredients of success, such as ongoing operational costs, construction requirements, cabling for new computers, licensing fees, maintenance fees, additional equipment needed, or increased staff needs. Particularly in technology areas, the clock on the warranty and maintenance coverage often begins ticking when the software or hardware is delivered, not when it is fully functional. Given the long lead-time of a technology project, the hospital may be paying for maintenance on a system that is still being implemented. Negotiating a contract that forces the provider of software to support the application until it is fully functional according to the mutually agreed upon specifications is possible, but takes a seasoned businessperson to achieve this in contract negotiations.

Consultants base their recommendations on what they believe can add value, but in order for this value to be measured over the long term, every major initiative should be required to present the following five items throughout the course of the project and subsequent to the completion of the project:

1. Business case
2. Budget
3. Schedule
4. Scope of the initiative
5. Performance against original target in all of these areas

The challenge is that some organizations will allow projects to drift into the future with no milestones identified, and because they are a pet project of a key political internal associate, they are allowed to get away with this behavior. Even the role of the corporate compliance officer can be compromised if they are a member of the organizational management team and dependent upon colleagues from other departments across the institution to provide them services. People at much lower levels in the organization would not be so lucky.

The budgetary confusion that consultants bring into the mix is often caused by their limited understanding of hospital operations, budgeting processes, and the differences between budgets built around a hospital census and those that are fixed expenses. Often hospital support departments are responsible for delivering services to areas outside of the in-patient area, and the requirements of these areas are continuous, regardless of hospital census.

These areas may include the engineering department, the IT department, the help desk, telecommunications, and the environmental services department. This complexity in the preparation of the budget creates a challenge when attempting to benchmark against other organizations and requires a deep knowledge of the expectations of the hospital that is not only theory-based, but also which is based upon real world operational experience.

One factor that makes consulting attractive to hospital leadership is that consultants are ultimately committed to delivering an outcome that will please those that hired them and consultants can do this with little regard for the long-term impact on business relationships. If their recommendations are unsuccessful over the longer term, they will be gone and the programs will be discarded. The selection of these consulting firms should be done very carefully and vetted openly among key operational staff members who offer operational insights.

Few organizations engage the operational teams sufficiently to understand the depth of their knowledge of what works, what doesn't, and why. It is easier to place this responsibility on the shoulders of consultants who may or may not deliver the desired outcomes. However, all consultants are viewed as outsiders without an ownership stake in the processes they attempt to change. The hospital staff also views them with serious concern about the amount being spent on their services. Although senior leadership may try to keep this confidential, rumors about what is being spent are commonplace.

Operational experts from all levels within the organization are often overlooked because of the perception that they are protecting their area of responsibility. The challenge is to create an environment that encourages creative problem solving that brings people together for the purpose of evaluating an issue without a sense of judgment. An organizational process that creates a "think tank" where issues can be discussed and openly addressed without fear of retribution creates an environment of problem solving that is rare in hospitals, but when engaged in lieu of consulting firms or in conjunction with these engagements, they are wildly successful.

In an interview for *Health Care's Most Wired Magazine* in the winter of 2008, Elliot Sussman, M.D., CEO of Lehigh Valley Hospital and Health Network, spoke about how he has engaged his staff in a concept similar to this. He calls it "the wild ideas team." There is a structure to the process that affords people the opportunity to work together to solve problems that are challenging to the hospital. Employees from all levels within the hospital staff these teams. They address workflow, project development and implementation, as well as overall quality issues. The physicians are engaged in the process and, as a result, performance is very high when measured by physician and nursing acceptance of process changes such as are required with an electronic medical record or computerized physician order entry system. Hospitals are always looking for best practices in their organizations, but few have grasped the value of the involvement of the hospital staff in developing sustainable process change as well as Dr. Sussman has demonstrated.

Hospitals take great efforts to conduct periodic employee opinion surveys (EOS), and in some cases, elaborate action plans are initiated to improve these surveys because hospitals wisely understand the connection between the EOS and positive outcomes. The hospital workplace creates a heightened reality where employees face tragedy and death up close. They also see healing and hope up close. This environment will bring out the best and the worst in people. Involved leadership is essential to achieve the right balance and to assure successful outcomes. Leadership must also be engaged, willing to change, and ready to provide support to all members of the organization. An openness and willingness to acknowledge mistakes, no matter how severe, is the time when consultants can be brought into the process to bring about the most effective change—if their alliance is to a mission, not an individual.

Chapter 16

Compliance and Purchasing

How a hospital or physician makes large purchases may seem irrelevant to the average citizen on a day-to-day basis, but it is important that we all understand that the decision making and contract negotiations for the systems that will be used by the physician or nurse are factored into the overall cost of doing business. When these contracts are not rigorously scrutinized, there is significant risk that the hospital will pay inflated costs for systems that may or may not deliver as promised. Equally important, if someone has received personal benefits due to these contracts it is difficult for them to challenge the outcome and they are forced to defend a substandard system or application. Vendors have been known to include publication of articles under the negotiator's name, arrange speaking engagements designed to enhance their career, or to pay large consulting fees to employees who may not purchase a system, but who are politically positioned within an organization to force the purchase of a system. The outcome is that quality is not challenged and problems are covered up, but more importantly, these unethical behaviors drive up the cost of healthcare.

The Office of the Inspector General of the United States has strict regulations regarding the processes that must be followed in order for any organization to receive funds from the government. Many private companies and charities also require adherence to these policies as a condition of the receipt of payment/funding for a hospital or related entity. These guidelines and processes are in place to avoid the presence of "sweetheart deals" when vendors, suppliers, or consultants are given inappropriate access to decision makers in the organization. However, the auditing of these policies is very difficult.

Large purchases are often conducted using a request for proposal (RFP), which may or may not include comprehensive terms and conditions, including the right to audit the books of the responding company. Responding to a comprehensive and well-written RFP can be very expensive to the vendor and willingness to do so is compromised if they feel that the contract award will be given to the vendor that has had the most "face time" with the authorizing employee or officer of the corporation. Large purchases that are completed without an RFP are reasonably suspicious and have the risk of artificially inflating the cost of doing business for the hospital. It is imperative that any organization that is granted not-for-profit status be held accountable to adhering to the policies of the Office of the Inspector General and with their own published or unpublished policies.

In order to receive government funds from Medicare, Medicaid, or for federally funded research grants, the purchasing process in hospitals must be competitively bid or there must be supportable documentation that the purchase is for a "best in class" product/solution/service or the provider has a unique knowledge in performing a service. It is the responsibility of the "C-Suite" to ensure that there is 100 percent compliance to these requirements. To make this easier, there are large independent purchasing organizations called group purchasing organizations (GPOs) that are separate from the hospitals, but which are available to hospitals that are members of their organization.

GPOs will sometimes conduct a competitive bid and secure pricing for various products, thereby reducing the burden on the hospital of securing competitive bids and reducing the risk of malfeasance. Other medical organizations such as the American Hospital Association may conduct comprehensive due diligence on a set of products and vendors and make an endorsement, in an effort to help hospitals in their decision process as well. This is valuable because hospitals are a relatively small market for a wide variety of solutions and as such it is sometimes difficult to find sufficient vendors to conduct a valid competitive bid.

Anytime there is a deviation from this process, the requestor is required to provide documentation regarding the reasons. If the documentation is insufficient, any employee aware of the issue has a moral obligation to notify the department known as corporate compliance because there is significant risk of inappropriate and possibly illegal behavior in the purchasing process without these checks and balances. There may be some fear of reprisals for making such a report, so hospitals are required to have an anonymous "tip line" for employees or vendors to us in reporting perceived violations. These reports are supposed to be independently investigated. In one case, an employee reported a series of financial impropriety to the anonymous compliance hotline and learned the hard way that this is not always a successful model.

The employee in question was aware of purchasing decisions and contracts that did not meet the stringent requirements above and reported it anonymously. The employee was given a "secret code" to use when calling back to find out the outcome. The compliance hotline then contacted the hospital's Chief Compliance Officer who turned the issue over to the very person that was accused of improprieties to investigate. When the issue came to a head, the Chief Compliance Officer simply stated, "If we can't trust our [the accused] vice presidents, who can we trust?" The employee took the issue of retaliation to corporate compliance, human resources, and the CEO before finally choosing to leave a very unhealthy environment where the worker had previously flourished. The CEO took no known action and failed to guarantee that the reporting employee was protected from retaliation, contradictory to his own publicly stated position.

This is important to the patient population because it establishes the ethics of the organization. While the organization in question may be inherently ethical, employees and leaders with low ethical standards and who are given the authority to spend these large sums of money will just as likely make decisions that will compromise clinical outcomes or worse, withhold this information from the public. The actions of the "C-Suite" will have a direct impact on the veracity of any information they share publicly. To paraphrase the aforementioned compliance officer—if you can't trust the executives of the company, you can't trust the company.

This is also important because the reporting relationship of the "C-Suite" needs to be closely developed. If someone is assigned the role of conducting an independent investigation into issues that are raised, then that person should not be someone with a supervisory or leadership relationship with the employee(s) or procedures being investigated. If there is a conflict of interest in the investigation procedure, the investigation will be compromised. A comprehensive conflict of interest questionnaire provides a false sense of security and will only reveal any of these conflicts when the person is honest. A dishonest person would have no qualms about lying on the conflict of interest questionnaire.

Another area of risk for financial impropriety is the activities of the political action committees (PACs), some of which have been documented in the media. News reports have the amount raised by political action committees on behalf of hospitals, insurance companies, HMOs, pharmaceutical companies, and physicians at more than $2.6B ($2,600,000,000). Many PACs were created for the purpose of giving the "little guy" a voice in government that is heard with sufficient clout to initiate governmental and policy change. Unfortunately what happens is that the PACs begin to have a life unto themselves and rather than serve a group of people, they serve a community of business interests with goals that may not be in the best interest of the public.

A CEO may choose to track the contributions of his/her executive team and then have them contacted by a colleague to follow up if the team hasn't made their annual donations. The underlying message is clear, so the contributions continue to roll in, whether you agree with the organization's goals or not. The objective of which is to influence legislation, gain government support for goals, or to ensure a favorable interpretation of a law.

Chapter 17

Legal Obligations

The Health Insurance Portability and Accountability Act (HIPAA) was conceived to ensure that people are able to purchase health insurance when they change jobs, voluntarily or involuntarily. HIPAA also includes extensive guidelines defining what is confidential or "protected health information." Approach any hospital employee about the purpose behind this bill and more often than not you will be told it is to protect patient confidentiality. They are less familiar with the primary reason behind the law—to secure continuing coverage when circumstances change. For details on HIPAA, access this website: http://www.hhs.gov/ocr/hipaa.

Another important law is the Emergency Medical Treatment and Active Labor Act (EMTALA). The interpretations of this law vary a bit based upon jurisdiction, but it includes language that stipulates that patients may not be involuntarily transferred from one institution to another unless the receiving institution provides a higher level of care. For example, a hospital without a neonatology unit could be forced to transfer distressed infants to another hospital. But unless the mother also requires a higher level of care, her transfer is not guaranteed, resulting in a separation of the mother and child. The mother's transfer would be considered a lateral transfer and the receiving hospital must have an available bed and a receiving physician who agrees to accept and treat the patient.

Under EMTALA, a hospital is required to respond to calls for emergency medical assistance using their own internal staff when the property is contiguous to the hospital. A building that is a block away, but connected by a pedestrian bridge, may be considered part of the "hospital," disallowing 911 calls for ambulance or paramedic assistance. They can be fined for calling 911 for medical assistance and these fines may be very large, depending upon the number of times it occurs.

In one case, a hospital provides outpatient services in space that is rented in a building next door and connected by a pedestrian bridge. The building is only partially occupied by hospital licensed clinical departments. In these areas, the hospital may not call 911 for assistance or transportation of the patient. However, if the patient is outside the door of the physician's suite, it becomes the jurisdiction of the city and 911 is called. It is nightmarishly complex and seems ridiculous, but this is an actual situation that existed in 2007.

EMTALA was enacted to ensure that the closest possible responder is legally obligated to act when a patient needs medical assistance. As it has been interpreted by some it just creates a quagmire of finger pointing and a burden on the hospital when the response isn't realistic. The law is interpreted in this way to avoid hospitals forcing high cost responses to other non-affiliated hospitals.

There was a very widely publicized case of a patient in the emergency room of a Los Angeles Hospital who was lying on the floor, vomiting blood, and could not get help because the staff of this hospital was inattentive (a janitor reportedly mopped around her, while she was writhing in pain on the floor). The family called 911, only to be told that 911 wouldn't respond because they don't respond to hospitals. Somewhere the concept of Do No Harm failed this patient and she didn't survive. Publicity around this incident and others at this inner-city hospital resulted in the closure of the hospital after the county was unable to turn their operations around.

The law does not prevent a staff physician or nurse from suggesting that the patient might want to transfer to another facility because of their higher level of expertise in an area. This happened to an associate who was hospitalized for a heart attack and needed surgery. The physician encouraged this uninsured patient to go to another hospital in the community to have the surgery because "the best surgeons were there," a reputation that was inconsistent with the message the initial hospital was promoting in their marketing plan. They were basically passing the buck because he was uninsured.

All of the preceding issues and regulations require each hospital to document their efforts to achieve their licensure and accreditation. While the physicians and nurses are documenting your care in your medical record, the remainder of the staff is certifying that all other forms of documentation are developed for support during accreditation, documentation in lawsuits, response to complaints, and to prove their contribution to the community they are identified as serving. People want to protect themselves and their careers; they aren't focused on the only purpose of a hospital that matters—*you*, the patient!

Chapter 18

Medication Errors

Medication errors are avoidable—even when the containers look alike and the names sound alike—however, the occurrence is significant enough to be dubbed "look alike/sound alike" risks. Studies have been conducted and the single most effective place to reduce medication errors is at the patient bedside, if the nurse follows the "five rights"—(1) right patient, (2) right route, (3) right dosage, (4) right time, and (5) the right medication. These are fundamentals of medication administration.

Most hospitals have P&Ps regarding specific tools or initiatives to avoid medication errors, but these policies should extend to when and how the patient or their family will be notified that such an error has occurred. Pharmaceutical companies have a responsibility to place medication in containers that are easily differentiated, with coloring or other design steps to ensure that they are easily distinguishable, but the simple truth is that a hospital may purchase medications from any number of pharmaceutical companies. Many of these medications are created in other countries like China, which is experiencing quality control and recall problems. It is unrealistic to think that the pharmaceutical manufacturers will all compare notes to decide how to manufacture distinct containers and medications.

Another type of medication error that is important to note is the absence of medication, particularly narcotics. The "absence of medication" refers to medications that are missing, stolen, misappropriated, or lost. Drug abuse is pandemic and hospital employees are not exempt. They have access to large quantities, knowledge of the effect of the medication and its practical application, and may lean towards self-medicating and self-diagnosing. They may enter that a patient was given a medication, but withhold it and save it for their personal use later, or worse, while they are on duty. The two most common tactics are (1) excessive wastage and (2) failure to deliver dispensed medication to the patient, while recording that it was delivered.

Dennis Quaid's family encountered a medication error that was a perfect storm of issues—look alike/sound alike medications, failure to follow the five rights of medication administration, and failure to validate that the correct medication was being placed in the correct bin in the dispensing location. In this situation Mr.

Quaid called the hospital to check on the twins and was told by the nursing staff that everything was fine. What the nurse didn't know or didn't communicate was that they had recently identified the medication error and that the children were seriously impacted. The hospital had a policy & procedure about medication confirmation, but not one about when and how quickly a family is notified of such an error. It also has not been established if the nurse that was held responsible was a permanent staff member or if that nurse had seen the medical center's policy regarding medication confirmation. Nor has it been established that the nurse's competency on the medical center policies was clear. Clearly the nurse and the pharmacy technician made a mistake, but where was the quality assurance process?

After a medication error occurs, the organizational wheels begin to spin, evaluating the situation from every possible angle. There is a meeting to investigate the occurrence, sometimes referred to as a Significant Adverse Event (SAE). The root cause analysis (RCA) is conducted to determine what changes in processes need to occur to avoid this error in the future. Hospital staff take these meetings very seriously. These are conducted in secret to some extent and result in substantive change by identifying avoidable negative outcomes and preventative steps.

There will be someone from risk management present. Lawyers, promising the confidentiality of the proceeding under "attorney-client privilege," usually staff Risk Management. The leader may announce to the participants that they are not to speak of the issue outside the room for risk of compromising "attorney-client privilege" as part of the peer review process. This prevents the meeting and discussions from being legally discoverable should legal action ensue.

Depending upon where you live and the resource pool that exists, many critical departments of a hospital may have employees that have a law degree. Human Resources is an excellent example of this, where they place people in charge of internal investigations and employee conflicts that have a law degree to assess the overall situation, validity of the issue, and the risk to the organization, while establishing attorney-client privilege, unbeknownst to those to whom they are speaking, particularly the complainant. It's a "just in case" scenario that some hospitals have adopted because of the availability of legal resources in the community. Risk Management, Human Resources, HIPAA Compliance, Corporate Compliance, executive committees, and boards may have attorneys present or part of the meeting, protecting the organization from exposure. This is not to say that it is standard practice at every hospital, but it is a technique used to mitigate risks when pockets are very deep.

In the proverbial perfect world, this wouldn't be necessary, but in a world where lawsuits are far too commonplace, it's not a bad strategy. The unfortunate thing about this practice is that important issues get blocked from public view. Things that should be corrected, and if not corrected, subsequently exposed are more easily hidden from public access.

When the RCA/SAE has been conducted, there may or may not be action items and it is usually emphasized that per accreditation guidelines the investigation is being conducted in a "blame free" environment, and employees are encouraged to speak and report issues. In many cases this is where conflicts in the P&Ps are discovered, confusion among staff about who is assigned particular roles in various situations are identified, and areas where clarification for the staff is needed are acknowledged. Unfortunately, what doesn't often happen is the hospital communicating the outcome of this to the patient or their survivors. On those rare occasions where the information gets out, the public relations machine will kick into high gear and a statement is issued along the lines of, "We prefer to keep our discussions on this very private matter between us and the family involved." Translation: "we don't want anyone to know about this and we want to minimize our exposure."

From your perspective, what you have to decide is why you want to know what happened. If real, lasting damage was done that will result in loss of income and/or increased expenses, you may want to contact a lawyer. Our personal belief is that it shouldn't become a legal matter unless negligence has occurred, if the event was foreseeable, or caused by staff members that shouldn't be treating patients. This last part gets really tricky because hospitals will correctly tell you that they cannot disclose confidential personnel issues that surface now or later related to the staff involved. Disclosing confidential personnel information is a risk to the hospital, but placing your life in the hands of a doctor or nurse that has problems that have been identified by hospital management should legally trump this right to privacy. Equally important, hospitals should track these situations and the personnel involved to see if any trend is identified. I am only proposing that active participants in the patient's care should be monitored for involvement in these major events to see if there is a staff member with challenges that aren't obvious to their immediate supervisor.

If your interest is to make certain that this event was a true anomaly and won't recur, then there is reason for you to know the outcome. Unfortunately, hospitals have no way of knowing who wants the information for what reason and so they "circle the wagons," minimize their own risk, and hopefully take the necessary steps to avoid these horrific experiences in the future. What it really comes down to is that in order to create an open environment where the hospital and patient can correct errors that slip by unnoticed, staff have to give up some privacy rights and the patient community has to be willing to be far less quick to litigate, leaving that only as a very last option after an internal review has been conducted. If your goal is a witch-hunt to get rid of people or receive compensation because of the mistake, then you may expect the wagons will continue to circle up and the system will continue along this dangerous path.

Chapter 19

Infection Control and The Environment

Hospitals are a great incubator for germs, it's sort of like a germ resort and spa. Protecting you from these germs is the responsibility of everyone in the hospital— patients, staff, and family members. As we saw in the aftermath of Hurricane Katrina, hospitals without power and air conditioning or heating can be death traps. The lack of air circulation creates a breeding ground for germs. Envision germs as passengers on a trip and their goal is to get as far as possible. A layover on their flight is nothing more than resting on your hands until you come in contact with the next person or thing.

In nearly twenty years working in and around hospitals, I never recall a time when there wasn't some sort of construction underway in the hospital. In fact, much of the work I have done has been in planning the delivery of information technology to these areas when construction was completed, which required involvement beginning with the planning stages of a remodel or new construction. Regardless of the type of construction, when a ceiling or wall is opened it releases a torrent of germs. These germs often have no impact on someone who is well, but for any patient who is immune suppressed—with cancer, transplant, Lupus, etc.—these germs can be fatal. Following along the Germ Journey, someone walking through an area where these germs are released (or exposed) may pick them up and unwittingly pass them along to another person and that person can pass them along to you. The germ gets quite a trip.

When a technician comes into your room to repair your television or replace your telephone, or a nurse pulls in a cart with a computer on it—all of these become ways that germs can get into your hospital room. The hospital has an ongoing obligation to ensure that the environment is as free as possible from the risk of infection. To that end, many hospitals have adopted a policy that identifies the procedures for authorizing work to be done in the hospital. Enforcing these policies may offer quite a challenge.

The transmission of these germs has an added cause and that is in the design of the space. Hospital personnel are amazingly creative, they have learned to make whatever they have work, and so if they don't have enough sterile or clean storage, they innovate. For instance, baby formula may be kept in a closet under a sink. If that sink leaks or has condensation on it, it could result in tainted formula. Or if the custodial staff doesn't have anywhere to put a mop and broom, they may put it in the closet that houses the equipment for computers and phones. Stretchers and wheelchairs are anywhere you can find one and you may be certain that they are stashed in some of the most obscure areas of the hospital, and guess what, they are conductors for bacteria as well, perhaps more so because they are in unsanitary areas.

When an architect designs space that overlooks the requirement for storage or makes operational assumptions about where things will be kept in a hospital environment that isn't consistent with the operational reality, the staff is forced to find ways to "make it work" regardless of local regulations or guidelines. Visits by the accreditation surveyors or the local fire marshal may result in a mad dash to move things around so the hospital is in compliance with these regulations. I've never seen a hospital nursing station or nursing unit with too much storage and someday I hope to see just that. However, I have seen them with inappropriately used storage and too much junk that is saved "just in case."

Although consultants and executives don't want to acknowledge it, every hospital is different. Priorities and risks shift from community to community, even when the hospitals are within blocks of each other. A functional design template is needed at each hospital to ensure the environment meets the needs of the staff and patients. Before demanding compliance with their vision, the hospital leaders need to find out from the staff what issues they face, then consult with the various support areas, such as information technology or information systems, housekeeping, food services, materials management, and security to determine their needs. Initially you will find that the staff members are afraid that this reality-based approach is not going to be sustained and they will overcompensate in their planning, but when hospital leadership demonstrates a strong willingness to collaborate, they will be surprised at the transformation throughout the organization. The number one priority is the patient care areas.

Numerous studies have been conducted into the risk of patient falls during a hospital stay. There is sufficient evidence to support the risk of patient falls to warrant that they be tracked by the hospital management as a core measure of patient safety. There have been recommendations that assistive devices such as canes and walkers be available to patients who routinely use these when not in the hospital. However, even the most agile of persons is compromised when in a hospital. It's a new environment, they are sick, they are probably weak, and they are on medication, making even the simple task of walking to the bathroom a potential risk of falling. A study by Washington University Medical Center indicated that "patients were injured in 42 percent of the calls," and "8 percent of the incidents caused serious injuries such as head traumas and fractures."

Many patients in a hospital are at least partially ambulatory. These patients may feel that they are capable of walking unassisted to the restroom in the middle of the night or they might just not want to bother the nursing staff. The worst-case scenario is that they are unable to reach a nurse for assistance and choose to walk on their own rather than continue to wait for help. Accreditation surveyors should consider evaluating the response to a patient call light based upon the time passage before a nurse enters the room. The information can be made available in most nurse call systems.

Have you ever looked around a hospital room? At night, the lights are dimmed, the atmosphere is much quieter, and the staffing of the hospital is lower due to a perception of reduced demand. Furthermore, being independent is important to most people. If a patient thinks they can move about without disturbing others, they will and it is likely they will get up and try to walk to the restroom. Depending upon the acuity of the patient, they may be tethered to an IV pole, there may be chairs in the room that are left over from earlier visitors, their bed tray may be in the way, any number of monitors may be in the way, and then there are all the cords everywhere— the electrical, the phone, their cell phone charger, etc.

The staffing has often been reduced and therefore the timeliness of a response to a nurse call light used to request assistance might be slower. The staffing reduction is designed to keep costs down. Perhaps hospitals should look at having a different lower level resource such as an "attendant" who serves as a force multiplier for the nursing staff and assists patients with these types of requests when an RN or LVN is not readily available. Hospitals should have a firm policy that the nurse call monitoring station is never abandoned, even for a few minutes, because if a patient needs to get to the bathroom, they will go if there isn't a response to their request for help in their own acceptable time frame.

We don't always communicate our sense of urgency and many of us were taught not to "bother the nurses and doctors." The outcome can be a fall due to design and overcrowding of an area, and that fall may result in long-term complications. Responding to the requests for assistance, medication, etc., should be a priority that is equal to the other predetermined orders that are pending, but hardly any hospitals can recruit enough nurses or other staff to meet the demand of the patients.

Few hospital rooms are spacious, unless you get a "deluxe suite." Architects will benchmark the price per square foot of construction against other projects where people previously made compromises, resulting in shrinkage in the size of the room based upon an expectation that a nurse or a nurse's aide will "manage the clutter" in the room, when they are already stretched to the limit. Furthermore, the benchmarking and costing data may be based upon a design of a building that was created five or ten years ago. The timing from conceptual design to completion of construction can easily be five years or more, meaning the design is outdated by the time the building or remodel is finished.

Creating designs that are functional, which address the risk of falls is possible, but it requires allowing the experts into the in-patient area to have significant say in the design. The construction of a mock-up room would also be beneficial. Every major hospital should consider a relationship with architectural schools to build relatively inexpensive mock-ups of patient rooms and nursing stations. Virtualized versions of the environment may work, if the nurse gets a real perspective of the area as it would be with a patient in the room, but from my own experience, the most successful approach is the construction of a model room, fully furnished and equipped. The furniture and equipment don't have to be fully functional, but it should address the line of sight from the patient room to the nursing station, nurse call visibility, and any safety or security issues of importance.

Chapter 20

Gateway to the Hospital

You may think that the information saved about you and your health status is only used for your treatment history, but the information has an inherent value to hospitals where it is often used in a variety of ways that might be unknown to the patient. After stripping out identifying information, the data is gathered from multiple systems. It is often used for data mining and is particularly valuable in medical research. However, it is also used for running cost studies or to develop a cost-benefit analysis of particular areas often called "service lines" or "centers of excellence" (COEs). For example, if a major not-for-profit healthcare organization were to conduct an analysis of their patient database, they might find that their emergency department is responsible for the largest number of uninsured admittances to the hospital. That information might have a direct relationship to any number of other operational issues. The funding to expand an emergency department that is only going to bring in more uninsured patients would not be justifiable from a financial point of view. Even the decision regarding whether or not to keep the emergency department open could be affected.

Of course, their ability to meet the demands of the community because of their altruistic mission isn't factored in. Perhaps it would be meaningful to start with minimal service requirements for all not-for-profit healthcare entities. If they are going to be given significant tax breaks, shouldn't they have accountability to their local community for the scope of services they do or do not provide? Equally important, as communities we must find effective ways to remove the non-emergent patient load that results in emergency rooms being used in lieu of having health insurance—by law, patients can't be turned away if they walk in!

Another significant factor impacting the business of healthcare is a growing trend for the more profitable "service lines" or "Centers of Excellence" (COEs) to be stripped away from the hospital by attending physicians who create small, boutique hospitals that focus on the patient population with a clearly identified ability to pay. To be fair, these decisions are more complex. The physicians often want a chance to make operational decisions exclusive of carrying the burden of less profitable lines of business. They often are focusing on a truly outstanding level of care for their patients, which sometimes puts the less profitable areas at risk. I found it interesting that five different department heads at my most recent hospital told me that their department was responsible for one-third of the revenue of the hospital. Obviously, each area felt they were critical to the life of the hospital, but the truth is that every department is critical to the life of the hospital, and every hospital is critical to the life of each patient. The trend of pitting for-profit healthcare against not-for-profit healthcare and the resulting mixture only serves to exacerbate an ailing healthcare system for the unemployed, the disenfranchised, the chronically ill, and the elderly. These patients rarely see the inside of a boutique hospital.

There are any numbers of personal, political, and/or operational reasons why physicians break off and create their boutique hospitals. One of them may be funding for research projects. Let's say a donor wishes to give a large amount of money to a hospital for research. I always thought that 100 percent of the money was going to the area of research identified. What really happens is that it goes into the budget, but then overhead expenses are taken out. What are these? Electricity, cleaning services, space utilization, utility bills, groundskeeping, staff support, paper, and other overhead costs of the organization. The inability to keep 100 percent of these donated funds for research purposes can be very upsetting to the individual physician researcher.

The great majority of Americans take it for granted, but 47,000,000 people in the United States remain without insurance. Their safety net is non-existent and they could have their economic future destroyed by a car accident, a heart attack, diabetes, or cancer. When they need medical help, they may decide to go to a clinic, self-medicate, or show up at the hospital emergency room. We have laws in place that prohibit turning them away from emergency rooms until their condition has been evaluated and stabilized.

The emergency room is the right place for the seriously ill or injured to be seen, regardless of their ability to pay. However, the emergency room is not the place to go for a routine physician visit when you have a minor illness or cold. The creation of a community-based safety net that is available to everyone in their own neighborhood—and where the quality of care is just as good in poorer neighborhoods as it is in the wealthier ones—is essential.

The reasons you may find yourself as a patient in a hospital will vary. It may be that you have been in an accident and transported there via ambulance, friend, or co-worker. You may have suffered a heart attack on the golf course. You may just be having chest pains and decide to walk in. Maybe you are there to have a baby or perhaps receive treatment for a severe or chronic condition. Regardless, you want the staff assigned to your care to be responsive and fully focused on your needs. It's OK to be selfish when you are the patient.

Most of these gateways into the hospital are routine. However, the enactment of the Emergency Medical Treatment and Active Labor Act (EMTALA) has changed one of these substantially—the emergency room. EMTALA rules have been revised on several occasions to provide further clarity and were initially enacted as part of the Consolidated Omnibus Budget Reconciliation Act (COBRA) of 1986, and Section 1867(a) of the Social Security Act.

People who are injured or who suddenly become seriously ill are brought to this part of a hospital and then perhaps admitted, depending upon the severity of the issue that caused them to seek help. Unfortunately, due to the absence of healthcare coverage for one-seventh of our population, these sites have become alternative locations to receive treatment that may have been avoidable if the health concern had been addressed in a more timely manner, or if preventative or interventional measures had been taken earlier. Part of the logic behind the Emergency Medical Treatment and Active Labor Act (EMTALA) was to prevent hospitals from refusing to see patients who are unable to pay.

Unfortunately, as with many legal reforms, the Act has been used to force hospitals to provide routine medical care, driving up the cost of healthcare for everyone, but more importantly forcing the temporary closure of emergency rooms when they reach capacity. Overcrowding in the emergency room or in the hospital results in more than 56 percent of ambulance traffic being diverted or rerouted to other emergency rooms each year. The traffic is redirected to the nearest open emergency room. Hospitals have a limited number of beds, a limited amount of staff, and the requirement for monitoring and staffing is dependent upon the acuity of the patient. If the hospital is full, but the emergency room is still seeing patients, overcrowding and delays will occur. If these patients are to be admitted, they have to have a bed, nursing staff, medication, physician oversight, etc.

The effect of the laws that mandate accepting walk-in patients even when closed to ambulance traffic effectively turns the emergency room into a doctor's office where those without an ability to pay may go to receive care, regardless of urgency. If the closures are because ERs are at capacity—and they routinely run at capacity—do the hospital ERs have an imperative to the community to expand that capacity or is there a different operational model that would off-load the non-urgent traffic.

One way of addressing the shortage of emergency rooms is to help change them back to their original purpose, instead of operating as the safety net for the uninsured or for those who can't get a doctor's appointment through their HMO. The creation of community-based urgent care facilities has been a successful model in some areas to help offload the patient volume to some degree, but does the law mandate the same care at these clinics that it does for a hospital? Perhaps not-for-profit entities or teaching hospitals should be required to establish off-site urgent care clinics that are geographically dispersed throughout the community and which are certified under the hospital's license. Providing a single standard of care would be the priority. This might meet part of their obligations under the not-for-profit tax code and solve the emergency room crisis.

Staffing these clinics is another opportunity for innovation that hospital leaders could champion. The medical field is changing at a pace unlike anything we've seen in generations. Perhaps requiring service for a year in an urgent care clinic should be part of the residency or internship for medical professionals. It could be tied to additional training for use of medical technologies that are being implemented in hospitals around the country. This part of a medical professional's internship or residency might be tied to the hospital where they are seeking to be credentialed, particularly if these clinics were hospital-based. There are many different funding models for these clinics. At a minimum hospitals that have been granted a not-for-profit status and the related tax breaks, should be required to spend a proportionate amount of money funding community based clinics and implementing new technology.

The business of the hospital above all else is to take care of patients, families, and colleagues. Hospital executives sometimes get the goals and the mission of a hospital confused. The strongest mission statement of a hospital is the simplest—to care compassionately for our patients as though they were our greatest love. In the absence of the ability to do that, the hospital should shut their doors. No meeting, no goal, no project is more important than treating those who have been entrusted to their care. This applies to everyone in the hospital—from the hospital's telephone operator through the CEO. If staff can't provide assistance, they are obligated to stay with that patient until proper attention is available. Finding new and creative ways to address the emergency room crisis is a fundamental issue that must be solved if we are to resolve our overall healthcare coverage crisis.

Hospitals are very hierarchical by nature. In many areas there are clear delineations between the role of nurse, physician, technician, pharmacist, and phlebotomist, to name a few. Nurses may be categorized into a variety of different levels, with different responsibilities or skills, such as LVNs, RNs, nurse practitioners, or nursing supervisors. Physicians have their own pecking order—interns, residents, senior residents, house staff, attending physicians, chiefs, and chairs.

Among physicians there is a value perception that has its own hierarchy based upon the area of specialization. This value perception often determines how they treat others. The role of a neurosurgeon may be considered the ultimate role of a physician, although a cardiovascular surgeon might disagree. Radiologists seem to be the Rodney Dangerfields of physicians because their role is not perceived to be in the middle of the action. These are all doctors with extensive training in their specialty, but medicine does lend itself to a very hierarchical operational style. The importance of a radiologist will become apparent when your MRI is reviewed and a diagnosis is accurately or inaccurately rendered. Remember, Rodney Dangerfield was a star too.

Every area in the hospital is filled with a variety of positions that are designed to use the appropriate skill mix to optimize performance and price. These positions provide supervisory oversight, continuing education, hospital policy guidelines, etc. But beyond these areas, we've all heard the term "hospital administration" which is where the big decisions are made and quite a few smaller decisions as well. Regardless of the altruistic nature of hospitals, they are still a business, employing a chief executive officer, chief operating officer, chief financial officer, chief medical officer, chief nursing officer, chief compliance officer, and now the chief information officer. This "C-Suite," as hospital administration may be called, is responsible for setting the administrative and clinical policies of the organization and is ultimately responsible for the operations of the hospital. Their management style will determine the outcomes experienced by their staff and patients. Despite the protestations to the contrary, every member of the "C-Suite" contributes to the individual medical outcomes and they should carry this responsibility cautiously.

Chapter 21

Accreditation of Hospitals

Hospitals that receive federal or state funds or federally funded research grants are required to submit to periodic surveys by an independent team of healthcare professionals and experts in various areas. These surveys are most commonly conducted by the Joint Commission for the Accreditation of Hospital Organizations (JCAHO). They are conducted at random intervals to measure adherence to internal policies and procedures, as well as to ensure proper proactive steps are being taken to address risks to patients and employees.

All responsible members of the staff take the accreditation surveys very seriously. The surveyors change their methodology for conducting their analysis from time to time and most recently are using a random patient's chart to follow their journey through the hospital. The surveyors may speak with anyone they encounter during their review—patients, family member, housekeepers, hospital operators, computer technicians—anyone they see. The joint commission and other accreditation bureaus have modified their approach to allow for more spontaneous surveys, but the hospitals still take the extraordinary efforts mentioned herein to make sure the surveyors see what they want them to see.

Some hospitals go so far as to tell employees who do not have urgent business in the medical center to stay away from clinical areas during the time the surveyors are there. Some hospitals take extraordinary steps to prepare for their survey, conducting mock surveys, reviewing all practices, and hiring expensive consultants to assess their readiness. When the surveyors arrive, they are assigned a place to work and are frequently escorted throughout the organization, somewhat controlling their access. Calls are made to notify areas if a surveyor is headed in their direction, e-mails are sent to alert staff of the course being followed. Hospitals communicate with their peers to find out what types of questions are being asked so that they can be fully prepared. The efforts to guarantee that the hospital does not receive any "Type 1" recommendations are significant. A Type 1 recommendation is a serious deficiency in the hospital and requires rapid corrective action.

A significant component of the accreditation survey is to assess the medical center's preparedness for atypical and unforeseen events that might otherwise compromise the ability to deliver care. The surveyors are given access to medical information, systems, charts, results, procedures for conducting peer reviews, your medical records, and any other issue they deem appropriate. An important aspect of access to medical information is the disaster recovery plan. This is a plan developed to identify how information would be recovered in the event of a catastrophic loss, such as what happened in New Orleans in the aftermath of Hurricane Katrina. During the Northridge earthquake in 1994, the water pipes above the medical records area of one hospital ruptured, soaking the paper. The staff undertook Herculean efforts to recover as much of the paper as possible.

However, the more common issue in a medical center isn't the major disaster that wipes out all electronic information, it is the network outage or downtime that prevents access to critical information when the needed information is time sensitive. Reviewing the hospital plans for ensuring maximum network uptime in both the voice and data areas is as important as disaster recovery, particularly as hospitals move towards a combined voice and data network, and place more and more of the essential information in electronic format. Equally important is the establishment of common definitions for what this "uptime" is and how it is measured. One person may define "uptime" as the time the application is unavailable, the network is unavailable, or the computer is out of service. Does it matter to you if it is the computer that the physician or nurse is using to try and access your medical chart? "Uptime" on a computer network may not result in the availability and accessibility of the information critical to your care, but if the "application" is up and devices used to reach them are not, does that have an impact on the clinical outcome?

When the Joint Commission for Accreditation of Hospitals Organizations (JCAHO) conducts their periodic surveys, they evaluate a wide range of issues to certify that proper infection control procedures are followed. They conduct a complete environmental survey, touring the most obscure of areas. This includes examining the physical firewalls that are designed to protect the occupants of a building in the event of a fire, checking water pressure, water temperature, air flow in isolation rooms, maintenance records for environmental systems, and making certain that the staff are conducting periodic preventative maintenance checks on these systems. They may check the nurse call lights, monitors, maintenance records for biomedical equipment, etc. The list of things they survey in the environmental areas is lengthy and comprehensive and is designed to secure a safe patient care environment. A similarly comprehensive survey of the information technology area still needs to be developed.

It is likely that there will be intermittent periods of unplanned system, network, or device outages that impact the accessibility of electronic information, which may impact your recovery. Will you ever find out that this was the cause? Unlikely. Common definitions for these outages have to be developed before true measurements are valid, then published in places that are easily accessible to the general population. An organization may win an award for being the most technologically advanced, but it is worth noting who provided the award. One popular technology award is currently affiliated with the American Hospital Association, but other awards may have affiliations that call their objectivity into question. Most importantly, a loose interpretation of the answers to questions may easily give an incorrect impression of an organization as technologically advanced, when the opposite is true.

Hospitals planning for these types of shorter-term emergency issues are usually covered in a business continuity plan that may be completely separate from the disaster recovery plan. These two very important plans may be under the responsibility of different members of the "C-suite." Business continuity plans focus on how the areas will operate when they are cut off from the normal information source or channels of information they use routinely. These plans should focus on ensuring network performance so that information is continuously available and what to do when there are intermittent, but longer outages.

One additional bit of information about joint commission—you, the community members, have the right to come forward and meet privately with the surveyors. Few people know this and fewer take advantage. If you believe that you have issues that should be heard by the accreditors, you should contact the hospital, ask to speak to hospital administration, and request the name of the accreditation bureau. When asking these questions, be sure to get the name of the person with whom you are speaking. If they do not provide you the information you requested, use an Internet search engine to find "hospital accreditation organizations" or "Joint Commission for the Accreditation of Hospital Organizations." Then give them a call or send a letter identifying your issue and request an opportunity to speak with them during the next survey.

It is important that your presentation be fact-based and supported to the extent possible to assure that your information is deemed credible. If you present action items to the joint commission, they are obligated to document, act upon, and respond to your concerns.

Chapter 22

Health Insurance - Paying the Bill

It is our challenge to lawmakers that each person's designated physician of choice should prohibit insurance companies from denying coverage for medically necessary care. The insurance company's policy of denial upon denial until the patient fights back, must be stopped legislatively since the industry has demonstrated an unwillingness to do so independently. Doctors often vary prescriptions and doses for different illnesses only to find out that the insurance companies only authorize a single large dose daily. Are there valid *medical* studies to support their conclusion? It seems that these deviations are strictly cost based, but they interfere with the clinical planning of the physician who knows the patient's condition and is aware of other medical challenges, yet cannot dictate the interval for prescribed medication.

Undoubtedly, there will be cases where the use of the phrase "medically necessary" is abused. However, the decision of whether or not a treatment or medication is medically necessary should rest solely on the shoulders of the medical professional responsible for our care, not on an arbitrary quota and not used for measuring physician performance. If there are cases of inappropriate use of this statement, it should be addressed in a peer review, with the results available to the public. It is the exception rather than the rule when a physician misuses the term "medically necessary" to provide superfluous medical care and they should have their license revoked. They are failing the first rule of care—*do no harm*.

Insurance companies should be allowed to evaluate inappropriate use of the phrase "medically necessary" after the fact and stop the victimization of the patient. A licensed physician should not have their recommendations overridden by an insurance carrier, regardless of their clinical training. Perhaps insurance companies should be subjected to surveys for accreditation, similar to those that hospitals experience, and these surveys should evaluate the number of times the insurance company denies care when a physician states it is medically necessary with full public disclosure of the outcome.

It is incumbent upon our legislators to establish that only the attending physician makes decisions about medical care and that insurance companies are not allowed to place restrictions upon the physicians, as they often do today. This is a legislative responsibility because insurance companies will very likely only make this change when legally required to do so.

Insurance companies should never have the right to limit our choices of physicians, our ability to seek a second opinion, or to create policies that delay care. Perhaps the Hippocratic oath should be applied to all involved in determining whether care is "medically necessary." The personal oath to "do no harm," whether by delaying care, denying care, or changing care must apply to everyone involved in the delivery of healthcare.

Insurance companies can deny claims for any number of reasons, forcing the patient or the provider into a series of appeals for coverage, or forcing the patient to pay in full, if they are able. Without knowing what information is administratively required to meet the insurer's test for medical necessity requires the patient or provider to try any combination of terms that will enable the insurance company to approve the procedure. In some cases, rather than be involved in the process, the provider requires the patient or their family to pay in advance of receiving medical services.

Anytime a patient seeks treatment they agree to certain terms and conditions, including a statement that they are required to cover any costs not reimbursed by their insurance company. Moreover, a doctor or hospital may then submit the claim to a collection company, who buys your bill for a fraction of the amount owed and then becomes your creditor. Sounds ugly. It is. This can result in damage to your credit while you are trying to find the right key word or phrase that will convert your claim from elective to medical necessity. This practice has to be stopped. According to Dr. Sanjay Gupta of CNN, nearly 50 percent of bankruptcies in the United States are the result of the costs of medical care.

Many people don't learn until it is too late that their medical insurance has a lifetime limit. In cases of major surgeries, with complications, extended hospital stays, or the ongoing requirement of nursing assistance, this amount may easily be reached before you know it. A day in ICU can run from $30,000 to $50,000, depending upon the type of care being provided. A surgical case may be more than $100,000. Once your carrier has paid the maximum benefit payable, you are on your own. The net result of this is that you may be forced into bankruptcy; you may lose your home or your ability to make a living. All of this at a time when you and your family are already at their most vulnerable.

Real Life Examples

Example 1

A patient experiencing severe chronic back pain caused by deterioration of their discs and complicated by scoliosis was approved for surgery and then experienced an unforeseen medical setback, extending their time in the ICU. The patient was diligent in confirming that his insurance carrier preapproved their surgery and conducted "in network," but while in the hospital, the physician used an anesthesiologist and other specialists that were not part of the "network" plan. The insurance company says that the charges for these services would be based upon using a provider that is "out of plan"; this drove up the co-pay, despite the insured's best efforts to follow the rules of the insurance company. The patients are often left holding the bag and if they want to fight it, they can look forward to massive delays, mounting legal bills, and years of continuing pain or death. Just the time on the phone needed to start the appeals process—trying to reach someone who can understand the issues and address the problem—can be overwhelmingly frustrating. Some insurance companies may deliberately make the appeals process more protracted than it needs to be in hopes that the patient will give up before they are forced to pay.

Example 2

A friend had an emergency appendectomy and was rushed into the operating room. He was on the table for six hours. After suffering complications because of his delay in seeking treatment (caused by his concerns about a lack of health insurance), he was not given a very good chance to live. He had a long hospital stay and recovery. After arriving home, the bill for $80,000 quickly followed. Ultimately, his credit was severely damaged and he is still trying to recover financially, many years after the incident. Financial difficulties are like dominoes lined up for a fall—when the first one hits, the others may fall quickly if they are close together. How the hospital accounted for his treatment is dependent upon the creativity of the accountants.

Anyone on a fixed income can have their lives destroyed by such a situation, wiping out years of their own hard work. Just two weeks in a hospital, particularly in the ICU, can cost hundreds of thousands of dollars. In the back surgery case above, the patient was also the victim of an avoidable medication error, further exacerbating his condition. Do hospitals charge for medication and treatment when an error occurs on their watch? Sometimes they do. How will you know? Have you ever tried to review a hospital bill line by line? Good luck!

The cost of the hospital stay could wreck the American family that is living paycheck to paycheck. In addition, it could do irreparable damage to their credit history, making the dream of home ownership or just having enough money to feed the kids, unrealistic. Just ten days in ICU could easily cost between $300,000 and $500,000, and you would rapidly be closing in on the maximum lifetime coverage on your policy.

According to voicefortheuninsured.org, "46 million Americans are uninsured." The United States spends nearly $100 billion annually to provide uninsured patients with health services, often for preventable diseases or diseases more efficiently treated with early diagnoses. Fortunately, Congress passed legislation to ensure that even those with a preexisting condition can carry their insurance with them if they leave their job. What Congress didn't assure was that everyone who has left his or her job could afford to pay for this baseline of care.

Could it happen to you? If it does and you take months to recover, the bills could be piling up or already in the hands of a collection agency while you are recuperating or grieving.

Insurance: As It Could Be

Insurance companies have an important role beyond that of paying the bill. Their current roles are to identify quality matrices and to consult with physicians on standards of treatment, but companies cannot play the role of denying treatment for what the physician believes is medically necessary. However, if an insurer has issues with the appropriateness of medical services provided, it is their responsibility to address this with the provider and not put the patient's care on hold until it is approved. In addition, insurance companies have demonstrated substantial value by acting as the negotiator for reductions in the costs of medication and care. They should take on the role of helping healthcare practitioners keep the costs down by forcing pharmaceutical companies to reduce their profit margin or coercing software and hardware developers/manufacturers to provide a longer product life cycle and eliminate the practice of treating hospitals and physicians like any other business.

If they can be trusted to do so, insurance companies could lead research efforts regarding the efficacy of treatment protocols. Their databases would be a gold mine for researchers to examine and cross check with their own results. They have the opportunity to be leaders in medical research and pharmaceutical development, if they commit that health insurance is not a business risk model, but a fundamental human right. That might require more than many executives or boards are willing to provide, but it could change the future of humanity in ways that would reach centuries into the future.

It is incumbent upon the state and/or federal government to pass legislation that protects the credit history, home ownership, savings, and property of people who are unable to pay. This will not be easy because there will always be people who will use any new rules to "game the system" and avoid payment. Billboards are covered with signs advertising lawyers who are "here to help you," but who really are offering to teach you how to work the system to achieve a maximum payout. This is a risk we need to address, but at the same time, seeking required medical attention should never result in someone losing their home to pay their medical bills, forfeiting their children's college funds, or losing their meager savings. Perhaps Congress should enact a standalone "Medical Bill of Rights" detailing protective rights, which doesn't have earmarks or riders attached. Isn't the great beauty of our Bill of Rights the simplicity—that we are all created equal and endowed by our creator with certain inalienable rights, among these being life, liberty and the pursuit of happiness? Life, liberty, and the pursuit of happiness were not mutually exclusive; they are guaranteed to all of us and isn't part of the foundation of life good medical care?

The American Dream is about lifting people up, giving them their chance to be invested in the success of our country. Can it ever be right for someone to lose their home because of their medical needs? Aren't we better than that?

Chapter 23

Things you need to know

Things you need to tell your physician

When you walk into any physician's office, hospital, or clinic, you need to know two things: (1) why are you seeking treatment today? and (2) what is your medical history? The doctors and nurses need this information in order to make an accurate diagnosis, so walk in prepared with information that they may find useful. Here are some examples:

1. Are you taking any medications, prescribed or over-the-counter?
    a. What type?
    b. Dosage?
    c. Frequency?
    d. When did you last take any of these?
2. Are you taking any supplements?
    a. What type?
    b. Dosage?
    c. Frequency?
    d. When did you last take any of these?

3. Do you have any allergies, particularly to medicines and foods?

    a. To what?

    b. What was your reaction when exposed to this?

4. Do you currently use any type of drugs or substances, legal or illegal?

    a. If yes, when did you last use the substance?

    b. How frequently do you use the substance?

5. Do you drink alcohol?

    a. If yes, when did you last have an alcoholic beverage?

    b. In what quantity?

    c. How often do you drink?

    d. How much?

6. Do you now or have you ever smoked?

    a. If yes, how much daily?

b. How long have you been a smoker?

c. If you've quit, when?

d. If no, do you currently or have you ever lived with a smoker?

e. If you have lived with a smoker, how much exposure did you have? (i.e., driving to and from work/school, in the house, etc.)

7. Do you have any chronic conditions?

a. Heart trouble

b. Diabetes

c. Arthritis

d. Anxiety

e. Depression

f. Cancer

g. AIDS

h. Autism

i. Colitis or Krohns

j. Epilepsy

k. Post traumatic stress disorder?

l. Have you ever been the victim of a violent crime?

m. Have you been in battlefield environments?

8. Who is your treating physician for any of these or other conditions not listed?

   a. Name
   b. Address
   c. Phone number
   d. E-mail

9. Have you ever had any surgeries?

   a. What kind?

   b. When?

   c. Where?

10. Have you been hospitalized for any other reason? Elaborate.

11. Biological history (if known)

    a. Parents

    b. Siblings (full or half)

    c. Grandparents

12. Are you adopted? If so, do you have access to your biological family medical history?

This is information that should be available to any treating physician or other appropriate medical professional involved in your care, including the EMT with you in an ambulance. It could make the difference between life and death.

Another issue you need to carefully consider is the treatment that you will be given at the end of your life. This becomes more complex as your life unfolds. In the case of my cousin Joyce, she was emphatic that she didn't want to be connected to any type of life support, but she overlooked one thing—her lungs were severely damaged and she ultimately developed congestive heart failure. Her mind was still very active and she was an optimist, so when her lung failure became much more acute, she made the choice to be placed on a ventilator and to be given a feeding tube. She lived for three weeks, received constant visitors, dealt with financial wishes and called as many people as she could to tell them that she loved them. Although there was some suffering in the end, no one in our very large family would have wanted to miss out on these last few weeks.

We think of a "do not resuscitate" (DNR) order as something that is put in place when we aren't able to make decisions on our own, but the circumstances may be different than we anticipated. For this reason, every time you are admitted to a hospital, this is something that must be addressed. Our minds change, our opinions change, and we should be clear about our wishes. I know that Joyce's decisions were right for her, but another person might have made a different choice.

Things You Should Ask Your Physician:

1. Who will be providing your care? Get all of their names.

2. If your physician is providing your care and is unavailable, who covers for them?

3. Is the person "in network," if appropriate?

4. Will the physician use any "out of network" providers in the process of treating you?

5. What are the possible outcomes of the treatment?

6. What is their success rate with this treatment?

7. How might the treatment impact your quality of life?

8. Do your doctor and other care providers have any fiduciary interest in any pharmacological company, lab, clinic, hospital, or organization other than their private practice, which they are using in your care? If so, what is this? Will they provide alternatives?

9. If you are unable to speak for yourself and you or your family has designated an advocate, will the physician or hospital commit to contacting the designee as soon as practical should a medication error occur?

10. Will the physician and the hospital commit to disclosing any information regarding medication errors, personnel issues, or other errors that affected your recovery or the outcome and the course of corrective action?

Things That Your Hospital Should Tell You:

1. Does the hospital publish a score card and make this publication available to all patients that covers the following:

    a. Infection rates that occur after admission
    b. Returns due to infections after discharge
    c. Number of readmissions within seventy-two hours of discharge
    d. Outcomes for various surgical procedures
    e. Number of medication errors

2. Does the hospital commit to maintaining sufficient staff and monitoring of your needs to accommodate the needs regardless of time of day?

3. Does the hospital commit to making patient education readily available, on demand, both prior to procedures and prior to discharge?

4. Will the hospital commit to maintaining sufficient staff and monitoring of your needs to accommodate the needs regardless of time of day?

5. Will the hospital certify that credentialing of physicians and nurses will only be granted upon verification and testing that they are familiar with all appropriate hospital policies & procedures associated with the hospital in which you are staying?

6. Will the hospital certify that all staff has equal and easy access to policies & procedures and that annual review of these is certified and documented in a tested environment?

7. Will the hospital certify that disaster recovery and backup procedures are in place for all electronic medical records, imaging information, and other information resources that are used in the course of your treatment, directly or indirectly?

8. Are any system downtimes forecasted? This might include applications such as electronic health record, computerized physician order entry, nurse call, the phone system, power, etc. Where are these downtimes posted?

9. When planned outages are required, are these outages posted at all entrances to the medical center in sufficiently large letters to be seen from a reasonable distance.

10. If there is an unplanned outage while you are hospitalized, what will be the potential impact on your care?

Chapter 24

Life, Liberty, and Healthcare

Societies everywhere and in every century have grappled with how to provide for those who are less fortunate than others. The discussion about healthcare in the United States is a continuation of this debate. It is unrealistic to believe that we will solve this problem for now and for the future without it being a work in progress. Regardless of your current position on the issues, this position will change if you or those you love become the ones in need.

In 1965, President Lyndon Johnson successfully incorporated his approach to these needs by legislation that was to become known as "The Great Society." This legislation introduced Medicare for all citizens over the age of sixty-five and Medicaid to those who lived an economically disadvantaged life. I doubt that he envisioned that one downside to Medicare would be that doctors would refuse to take new patients that were covered by Medicare, but unfortunately, that happens everyday. The option of refusing to take patients who are covered through these programs, forces the burden of patient care onto the backs of those who understand their obligations as medical professionals.

Just as in the 1940s and again in the 1960s, we are faced with challenges to sustain the programs of the past and to expand them into the future. This occurs at a time when there is legitimate concern that funding for various social programs may cease to be economically viable. The survivability of Social Security, Medicare, and Medicaid is questioned by many and our deficit is at historical levels. Despite these challenges healthcare is frequently ranked among the most important concerns in each election process. Should the government intervene and provide universal healthcare coverage to everyone within our borders and risk breaking the bank or do we ignore the suffering of the disadvantaged in our country?

Our nation is at a crossroads and faces the challenge, the cost and the opportunity to provide healthcare to anyone in need; failure to do so is to deny the core values upon which our nation was founded. We must continue the investment in technologies and research and we must make these new treatment protocols available to everyone when they are deemed to be safe. The investments in technology will result in an ongoing financial demand for periodic upgrading and/or replacement through the life cycle of the technology. We must understand that this investment is essential to controlling costs, but will likely not have the effect of driving costs down.

We must provide access to healthcare in all of its forms by identifying further legislative and tax reforms for patients, families, hospitals, physicians, employers, and insurance companies. We must establish a timeline for incremental change and we must deliver on the words of poet Emma Lazarus as inscribed at Ellis Island to "Give...[us] your tired, your poor, your huddled masses...send these, the homeless...to me." Are we still the nation that aspires to form a more perfect union? We decide each day.

WORKS CITED

Abdollah, Tami. "Customers Acts Fast to Shore up Systems." Los Angeles Times. 4 September 2007: B1.

American Hospital Association. <http://www.aha.org>.

Committee on the Consequences of Uninsurance. Hidden Costs, Value Lost: Uninsurance in America. Washington, D.C.: National Academies Press, 2004.

Dotzour, Mark and Beth Thomas. "What Is in Your Building?" Tierra Grande: Journal of the Real Estate Center at Texas A&M University. April 2008: 6-8.

"Facts on Health Care Costs." National Coalition on Health Care. 5 June 2008 <http://www.nchc.org/facts/>.

"Frequently Asked Questions about the Emergency Medical Treatment and Active Labor Act (EMTALA)." 2 August 2008. <http://Emtala.com/faq.htm.>

Gupta, Dr. Sanjay. Chief Medical Correspondent. CNN. 2008

Home Page. Taxfoundation.org. 2 August 2008. <http://www.taxfoundation.org/blog/show/1295.html>.

Institute of Medicine of the National Academies. A Shared Destiny: Community Effects of Uninsurance. Washingon, D.C.: National Academies Press, 2003.

Lazarus, Emma. "The Colossus." The Poems of Emma Lazarus in Two Volumes, Vol. 1. Boston: Houghton, 1889.

Mintz, Jessica. "Windows XP's Fans Rallying to Rescue System." Austin American Statesman. 14 April 2008: D1.

Ornstein, Charles. "Footnote to a Tragedy." Los Angeles Times. 15 July 2007: A1.

Purdy, Michael C. "Hospital Falls Study Suggests Ways to Reduce Risk." Washington University in St. Louis, School of Medicine. 16 April 2008. <http://alladin.wustl.edu/medadmin/PAnews.nsf/PrintView/B6B3E706041D5BB86256EAF995AADE6?OpenDocument>.

Rubin, Joel. "District Payroll: A Lesson in Misery." Los Angeles Times. 25 August 2007: A1.

Runy, Lee Ann. "The Wild Ideas Team." Health Care's Most Wired Magazine. Winter 2008: 9-13.

Shapiro, Ellen, Champ Clark, Sharon Cotliar, and Susan Schindehette. "Coverage Denied." People Magazine. 23 July 2007: 64-68.

Smith, Andrew. "TI Aims to Change Medical Care with Smarter Chips." The Dallas Morning News. Austin American Statesman. 14 April 2008: D4.

Tanner, Lindsey. "Hospital Mix-ups Hurt Kids." Austin American-Statesman. 7 April 2008: A1.

"The Declaration of Independence of the Thirteen United States of America." United States. John Hancock, et al. 1776.

United States Department of Health and Human Services, Center for Disease Control and Prevention, National Center for Health Statistics. Summary Health Statistics for the U.S. Population: National Health Interview Survey 2004. August, 2006.

United States Department of Health and Human Services. 26 June 2008. <http://aspe.hhs.gov/poverty/01poverty.htm>.

United States Department of Health and Human Services. 26 June 2008. <http://www.hhs.gov/ocf/hipaa>.

"VoiceForTheUninsured." American Medical Association. 7 June 2008. <http://www.ama-assn.org/ama/pub/category/17712.html>.